WHEN NATURE'S
NOT ENOUGH

WHEN NATURE'S NOT ENOUGH

Personal Journeys through In Vitro Fertilization

BY DIANA M. OLICK

THE LYONS PRESS
Guilford, Connecticut

An imprint of The Globe Pequot Press

The Lyons Press is an imprint of The Globe Pequot Press.

10 9 8 7 6 5 4 3 2 1

Printed in the United States of America

Designed by Sheryl P. Kober

ISBN 1-59228-542-2

Library of Congress Cataloging-in-Publication Data is available on file.

For Scott, who honestly believes I can do anything...

And for Noah and Madeline,
finally a family

CONTENTS

YOUR PREGNANCY

KIDS!

ACKNOWLEDGMENTS

G iven the number of double strollers I see on the sidewalks of my neighborhood, I know that there are fellow IVFers in my midst. And for every person I tell about this book, they inevitably know one or two friends who have been through IVF as well. They say there is safety in numbers, but I'm not sure that applies here. Living through IVF is one thing, talking about it requires a whole different pool of courage.

To all the couples that shared their stories with me, I am eternally grateful. In the interest of clarity, I chose only five to detail in depth, but that certainly doesn't mean that the rest of you aren't there. Your wisdom, knowledge, values and strength are all included in this work, even if not your names. Without the many interviews, I would not have been able to find the many answers, nor would I have been able to understand all the facets of IVF from all the varied angles. This is a collaborative work of some truly extraordinary volunteers, and I never forgot that as I wove together their unique contributions.

One of those willing volunteers was Dr. Preston Sacks. About three years ago, I paid him to do a job, and he has been paying me back ever since. Never does a phone call or email go unanswered, as I bother him with issues technical, emotional and occasionally irrational. I have never met a physician like him and doubt I ever will again.

I would like to thank Martha Kaplan and Nicole Hirsh for their insights and more so for their perseverance. I appreciate their trust in my goal and ensuing support.

I would also like to acknowledge my editor, Ann Treistman, who believed in the value of this work right from the start and who helped me to focus when the profound emotions of this subject sometimes blurred my journalistic vision.

This book is as much for those who helped me as it is for those I hope to help.

INTRODUCTION

I'll never forget the day my gynecologist fired me. He didn't actually do it himself; he had his nurse do it. It seemed he no longer required my business. There I was, an early thirtysomething, healthy, married, financially secure woman ready to have children. What more could an ob/gyn ask for? Apparently, much more.

After six months of trying to conceive, my husband and I were starting to worry. Okay, panic. According to everything we read on the Internet, even under normal circumstances it could take up to a year, but deep down I felt something was wrong, so we headed for the gynecologist. He greeted us warmly, overflowing with all the consoling words and wisdom we were looking for. He even said that if there *was* a problem, which he doubted *highly*, we would "get through it together." But when I suggested we start some actual tests, he balked. When I begged, he more than balked. In what I can only judge in retrospect as a preemptive strike against losing a patient, he suggested that he knew our "type"—young, urban, ambitious couple that wants everything, babies included, to arrive exactly according to plan. Translation: you waited selfishly into your thirties, frivolously toying with your careers and your freedom, and now you're going to pay the price.

Was he right? Had I spent too much time indulging myself in whatever fancy came across my path? I was a television journalist, and when you're starting out in that career, you live on the end of a pager. I had traveled most of the country and a nice chunk of the world, responding, like an ambulance, to every flood, fire, hurricane, tornado, and human disaster in the making. I started when I was twenty-four years old, moved to eight cities in seven years, and had about five real dates during that time. I didn't get married until I was nearly thirty-three and only then, for the first time in my then five years as a CBS news correspondent, did I finally settle down to a less-mobile assignment in Washington, DC. My husband started a new business, and we bought a house with three bedrooms. We were ready.

Little did we know that no matter how much planning and preparing you do, getting pregnant isn't as easy as it looks on TV. Ironically, when I was single, I was always terrified that I would get pregnant. I was vigilant about birth control, and even then I worried if my period was a minute too late. So when things didn't happen as we expected, I immediately blamed myself. Was this the punishment for pursuing my dreams?

To call me overambitious would be an oversimplification. I was raised in New York City, the youngest of three, and the only daughter of two successful attorneys who clawed their way out of the Bronx and onto Park Avenue, but who still believed that nothing wonderful ever just happens. If you want something great, you'd better be prepared to work your ass off to get it, and even then it's not guaranteed.

They gave me a marvelous education and an invaluable trough of common sense, and they always taught me to protect myself by being prepared, smart, and careful. They had worked relentlessly to tear away from their poor Jewish roots, economically and socially, and even though I was raised in their resulting affluence, it never occurred to me that I shouldn't work just as hard as they did.

I wanted to be a network news correspondent, and patience is not exactly one of my virtues. I knew I had to slug it out in local news but didn't want to spend a second longer than I had to out in the boonies. So I raised my hand for every assignment and never took a day's vacation, and in two years and eight months, I got my first network offer. In fact, I got two. But the work didn't end there.

Starting at a network means starting at the very bottom and saying yes to any and every assignment, no matter how tedious or torturous it is. I often wondered, as I stood in the rain for hours or waited for another delayed flight or napped in yet another acrid rental car as some overcaffeinated producer pitched us across the heartland, why people think TV news is so glamorous. At my level, it was just plain tiring, frustrating, hard work. Still, the work paid off, and after a few years I was in a position to ask for some small things, mainly an assignment back in New York.

By then I had spent the bulk of my energies and my twenties running around, standing in front of satellite dishes, eating questionable foods in questionable strip malls. Were these the energies I needed to get pregnant? I thought about that one for a while. Then I beat myself up over it for a while. Finally, my glass-is-half-full husband convinced me to take a less emotional approach and check the facts. Unlike me, he came from a family that believed in all possibilities.

Scott grew up in Boston, the son of two ambitious, successful, extremely optimistic parents. His grandmother used to tell his father that he shouldn't try so hard to get out of the small Jewish neighborhood where he grew up, a neighborhood where most people had equally small aspirations. She told him he would only be disappointed when he failed. But Scott's father broke out and succeeded well enough to retire to an Arizona golf course at age fifty. He taught his son that anything is possible.

Scott's mother came from a deeply political family in New York City but found her real calling in Boston. She went to college and law school there, mixed it up in Boston politics as an assistant attorney general, was a regular in the local media, taught, wrote, and raised two children and a dog. She sees every door as wide open.

Even with all their work, Scott's parents are deeply committed to family, and despite the fact that they've been divorced for more than twenty years, are still great friends.

They gave Scott the mind-set that there are no wrong turns in this life, just new opportunities around each bend. Sometimes I find his optimism unrealistic, sometimes downright annoying. I certainly did in the case of our infertility. I didn't want to wait and expect the best, as he did. I wanted to attack.

After much prodding, my gynecologist agreed reluctantly to do a couple of hormone blood tests on me but suggested that testing my husband was premature. My tests all came back fine, so we waited. While we waited, we tried everything else.

First, those ovulation predictor kits from the local drug store. But they were hard to read, and I was never fully convinced that I was actually ovulating when the little white stick said I was. Then I decided to go high tech. I saw a commercial on television for a little computer that actually flashes an egg on the screen when it's time. One week later I was its proud owner.

We even took my mother's expert advice and planned an extravagant island vacation to coincide exactly with my ovulation. Getting rid of daily stress would certainly get rid of our problem. Three days into the trip, as I stood in the bathroom of my ocean-view bungalow, the little egg flashed on the computer screen! It was perfect— the sun, the palm trees, the romance hanging softly in the ocean air, and the gentle blinking of the little black digital oval. Well, the water was nice anyway.

But then I found the answer! One week on an island was a pitiful attempt at relaxation. If you want results you go to the professionals, right? And there it was in black and white: acupuncture. A few weeks after we returned from the Caribbean, I read an article in *Washingtonian Magazine* about a woman who had irregular periods and was having terrible trouble conceiving. After therapy with an acupuncturist, her periods came on time, and finally she got pregnant. The article suggested that acupuncture could stimulate certain hormones in a woman and thereby increase her fertility. It didn't actually sound so off-the-wall, even to overly skeptical me.

So I ended up in the DC offices of a very kind, very soft-spoken Chinese woman, who specializes in acupuncture for infertility. I went probably six or seven times, and while I guess I found it somewhat relaxing, being in a quiet room with soft music and dripping water from one of those plastic fountains, the more I spoke to her, the more confused I became. I would tell her about the noninvasive fertility procedures I had read about on the Internet, like artificial insemination, and I spoke quite confidently about my little egg computer. She just smiled and nodded but never seemed to offer any of the rah-rah spirit I was looking for. She frankly didn't seem all that encouraging. Then one day, I went to see her while I had my period. She could see I was feeling particularly dejected. For a moment, she looked uncomfortable, then paused, and finally said that while acupuncture would definitely help me spiritually and had been shown in studies to increase the production of certain necessary female hormones, in the end, most of her patients went through in vitro fertilization (IVF). I stopped going to her after she told me that.

By eight months, I was in a panic. According to my personal history, if I worked hard enough, I should get what I want, right? There was the work, where was the payoff? I called the doctor again and asked if he would test my husband. Again, he dissuaded while I pleaded. Finally he relented and gave me the name of a clinic where we could get a sperm analysis for about $90. Cup and credit card in hand, my husband headed for the little room all men dread. It wasn't too bad, though; this place even had videos, and my ever-optimistic husband was sure he was fine. This was just a formality to shut me up. Two days later, we learned we had a problem.

The urologist told us that with my husband's sperm count and motility, we had about a 5 percent chance of ever getting pregnant on our own. I immediately phoned my ob/gyn to deliver the bad news, but he was on vacation, so, as directed by his nurse, I faxed in the test results and waited a week. When he didn't call back, I called again. His nurse said he would get back to me that day. When he didn't, I called again the next day. After all, he had said we'd get through any problem "together," right? This time the nurse suggested that the doctor had other patients and plenty of paperwork on his desk, and I would simply have to wait my turn. I waited. The next day she called back and said she had spoken to the doctor, and he told her to tell me, "We simply can't help you." The nurse suggested we find a specialist and warned it could take months to get an appointment. "But," she added, "please do call us back if you get pregnant." Sure, I'll do that. I never even got to speak to the doctor.

That was it. Buh-bye. Good riddance. We were now on our own, facing the biggest problem either of us had ever encountered. We got no guidance, no words of wisdom, not even a consoling call telling us everything would turn out all right in the end. That's because there is no easy answer to infertility. There are clinics and doctors and options, but no guarantees and no one who is going to be able to say with any authority that it will actually turn out all right finally.

I don't mean to imply that all ob/gyns will react this way, but I know someone else who had the exact same experience. In fact, I have to give her credit. She was the one who called me one day in a rage and exclaimed, "My gynecologist just fired me!" I don't think everyone gets such a reaction, but in talking to other couples in this situation, I've found that many ob/gyns today are reluctant to even consider there might be a fertility problem before a couple has tried for at least a year. This leaves the infertile couple to wait, wonder, and worry alone, scanning books and the Internet, looking for some magic answer to reassure them that someday they will hold a bundle of joy. For many, that bundle of joy will take equal parts money, emotional anguish, and physical pain: they will choose in vitro fertilization.

I have to admit, I had never heard of IVF, and I've been a journalist for over a decade. I actually didn't do much research on it until I'd already done it. Crazy? Maybe. But because we had male-factor infertility—that is, there was nothing wrong with my plumbing—there were really very few options if we still wanted to have a baby that was genetically both of ours. We tried artificial insemination three times (it's called intrauterine insemination, or IUI, and I'll explain more about it later), but when that didn't work, there was really nothing else to try. Even though IVF has only a 25 percent success rate for a woman in her early thirties (it drops to about 5 percent in your early forties) it seemed far better than the 5 percent chance our specialist estimated, given Scott's sperm issues. In retrospect, it seemed like we were in this haze of need, wanting so much to get pregnant that we just did whatever our specialist told us to do. After three months of IUI, he said we could keep on doing it and maybe we'd get pregnant, but if we wanted to be "aggressive," then IVF was it. So we did it. I'd heard of test-tube babies, but that seemed like something very esoteric and very rare and almost disconnected from what we were attempting to do. I'll also admit, I didn't even know the *true* meaning of the word "infertility." I've learned a lot in the last three years.

Early on, a nurse in that wonderful ob's office told me that if I couldn't get pregnant in a year, that meant I was "infertile." *I* was infertile. Despite the fact that a 2001 congressional investigation found that infertility affects men and women "with equal frequency," she said it like it was all me, all my problem, and so I panicked, thinking "infertile" meant I could never ever get pregnant. Not so. According to the Centers for Disease Control (CDC), 7 percent of all married couples in America have been diagnosed as infertile, and that's just married couples. In 2001 (the most recent data available from the CDC) 107,587 assisted reproductive procedures (referred to in medical circles as ART), the vast majority of them IVF, were carried out and resulted in 40,687 bouncing bundles of joy. Infertile couples can get pregnant.

There are three types of ART procedures, but IVF, which has been improved in the last nine years, is the most popular and is only increasing in popularity as its success rates improve. In 2001, of all the ART procedures documented, 99 percent were IVF; that's more than 106,000 IVF procedures carried out in the United States in one year alone.

Still, when I first heard those three big letters, I had no idea what I was getting into. "In vitro" is Italian for "in glass." It's what they used to call test-tube babies, only now they do it in a dish. In 2001, 384 fertility clinics were vying for business in the United States, and there are estimated to be close to a million people walking around today who were conceived in a dish. It is big business, a billion-dollar business in fact.

We found a wonderful fertility specialist who sat us down for almost two hours and explained the procedure as something like this: using a complicated regimen of drugs, over the course of about six weeks, the doctor manipulates the female system to overproduce eggs. Just before those eggs would be naturally released by the ovaries, the doctor heads them off and retrieves them by inserting an ultrasound-guided needle through the vagina to the ovaries' follicles and removing the fluid containing the eggs. Then the eggs are introduced to the sperm in a dish and watched over the next few days for fertilization, that is, if the sperm and the eggs get together. Fertilized eggs (embryos) are then transferred into the woman's uterus using the same procedure as artificial insemination (often called "turkey basting"). The doctor uses a catheter to basically place them back in. How many embryos go back in is a tough choice and one I'll spend time on later, but that's a layperson's version of how it all works.

Our fertility specialist was really thorough in explaining all the many technical steps of the drug regimen, retrieval, and transferal, but as my husband and I embarked on what we now call this "mad science," we found very little in the way of personal narratives, stories of the many hurdles couples confront before, during, and after this process. Doctors will give you a dizzying array of statistics, pros and cons, but the choices are all yours, and there are plenty of them.

Right from the start, we realized how many misconceptions we had about IVF, and the more we told others about what we were doing, the more we faced their misconceptions of it as well. That's why we wanted so badly to be able to peek into someone else's window, someone who had already been through IVF, and see what they did.

The trouble is, infertility is not exactly cocktail-party conversation, even now. It is, however, slowly coming out of the closet. Singer Celine Dion and Brooke Shields made the cover of *People* magazine with their in vitro experiences and Lance Armstrong wrote in his best-selling book, *It's Not about the Bike*, that having his son through IVF was a greater victory than winning the Tour de France. Even the wildly popular HBO comedy *Sex and the City* tackled IVF in a story line, showing how one character's marriage could not survive the stress of going through the process.

Still, the average couple faced with a complicated fertility procedure tends not to discuss it with friends. In talking to other couples, I found that most people just don't want the extra pressure. Many said it was simply too hard to explain the whole procedure and then keep their friends and families up to date on the success or failure of each step. Others were ashamed of their inability to do what everybody else seemed to be doing so easily. Most just didn't want to be pitied or judged.

Nearly every step of IVF begins with a decision: if, when, how, and even why to start; what to expect emotionally from the choice; the drugs and the procedure itself; how many embryos to put back in after fertilization; what to tell family, friends and coworkers; the difference between a normal and an IVF pregnancy—to name a few. And then there is the stigma of IVF. The specialists will tell you there is no difference between a normal and an IVF pregnancy, but there is; IVF can create a sense of shame and fear. What will others think of what I did? Is it my right to mess with nature? Will my children really be normal humans despite what I did to create them? And don't forget about all the financial aspects.

IVF can cost anywhere from around $4,000 to $12,000 for just one try, and some couples will need to go through many cycles. As of 2004, only fifteen states require insurance carriers to cover some parts of advanced infertility treatments such as IVF; nationwide only 25 percent of all health plan sponsors provide coverage for infertility services. A federal bill in Congress that would require all health insurers to cover infertility treatments has been languishing since the spring of 2001 with little hope for passage.

Because IVF is now a multibillion dollar business, the field has obviously become increasingly competitive, and that can have some dangerous ramifications to the individual. It is in fact so competitive that some clinics are offering money-back guarantees if they don't get you pregnant after a certain number of tries. Just turn on your morning-drive radio, and you can't get away from all the ads. One of the more popular clinics in DC touts its "IVF Shared Risk Refund Plan" on the front page of its Web site. "One hundred percent Refund Unless You Have a Baby." The trouble with all the competition is that success rates of the clinics, which are required by law to be published annually, become their greatest marketing tool. Consequently, some doctors, not all but some, will pressure a couple to transfer more embryos in the hopes of upping the chances for success. This of course leads to a higher incidence of twins, triplets, and quads, high-risk pregnancies that can result in all kinds of complications to the children and the mother. We never considered any of this simply because we knew nothing about it.

It was only after we went through IVF that we began talking about it more openly. The more we talked, the more we heard stories of others who had gone through the same thing. We would mention it to another couple over dinner and then hear about how their friends had tried IVF four times or how another couple had tried to get pregnant for ten years. The more we talked, the more we heard and learned. If only we had talked before. That's when I decided to write these stories down.

I interviewed couples from varying economic, social, and religious backgrounds. These are regular folks, the kind who live next door. All of them have struggled with infertility, anywhere from two to ten years, and all of them ended up trying IVF, some successfully, some not. In an effort to get to the heart of the experience, I will focus mainly on five of these couples and follow them as they face each medical, social, and emotional step involved in IVF.

I also include my own experiences and the difficult physical and emotional aftereffects that many of the couples I spoke with shared but were more reluctant to talk about than the actual IVF process. Even successful stories don't always have the happiest endings. Some of the happiness is hard fought. New studies today show the emotional and physical stresses of IVF, coupled with high-risk pregnancies and multiple births, are creating difficult and sometimes dangerous results on children, parents, and marriages. These are also factors I wish I'd known about before I started. I don't regret what I did, but I regret being so poorly informed, and that's what I'm seeking to change with this work.

Hopefully, these stories will empower those embarking on this complicated journey with the experience and wisdom of those who have traveled the road before—and survived.

When Nature's Not Enough is not a medical resource; there are plenty of those publications at your local bookstore, many of them quite informative. I am a journalist, not a doctor. These are real stories of real people, like myself, facing a really terrifying and often puzzling process, a last resort, all in a desperate effort to have a child.

WHEN NATURE'S
NOT ENOUGH

Choosing IVF

CHAPTER 1

INFERTILITY

I never saw those two pink lines. To this day, I never have. In the beginning, that was the hardest part of infertility. Every month I would wait the allotted days and head for the bathroom, hoping, praying, *expecting* to see a positive result on this lame plastic pregnancy test. But I always came up short one line. I always came up short when it came to being like everyone else. That may sound trite, not too terribly deep, but those little white test sticks were larger than life to me, probably because they represented the possibility of life; in my eyes they gauged what was normal, so every time I got a negative result, I was suddenly some kind of deviant. I was a failure, not just as a baby maker, but also as a human being.

Reproduction is supposed to be the most natural phenomenon there is. If I couldn't do it, then somehow I didn't belong. I know everyone reacts to infertility differently, but I do think this is a common thread, the feeling that the inability to have a child somehow separates you from the human race as we know it. It's almost as if you were an extra in the big show but never allowed to play a real part. Put simply, you have no purpose other than to take up space, go through the motions, and never leave any real contribution to society. I know this sounds melodramatic; I get that. Of course there are people who choose not to reproduce. Some choose not to because they are too busy contributing to society, because they are so much a part of life that they simply don't have the time, energy, or inclination. But that's a choice. When your choice is to have a child and you can't, then the meaning of life takes on a whole new face. The meaning of society and your place in it changes drastically. You are simply not like everyone else.

As the months passed, my husband and I found ourselves avoiding our friends who had children, leaving bring-your-kids Christmas parties early, and even distancing ourselves from young nieces and nephews. We were at the age when everyone we knew was either having their first child or working on number two. The dialogue of our friendships was changing; it used to be careers, relationships, current events. Now it was babies. Having babies, caring for babies, registering for baby gifts, going to baby showers, burping, teething, pooping, potty training, ear infections, preschools, nannies, et cetera to eternity. We just couldn't face the fact that we weren't a part of what seemed to be, in our minds at least, an increasingly exclusive club.

I also began to feel like pregnant women were stalking me. Crazy, I know. Obviously it was a heightened sensitivity to my predicament, but that didn't make it any less real. First it was on television. Every other commercial was for a pregnancy test kit. I was sure of it. There was the nice young couple, holding the stick, waiting for that great result, and then they'd smile knowingly at each other, and through joyful tears coo, "We're going to have a baby!" Then the stalkers moved outside. Every day, as I walked the fifteen minutes from my news bureau to my home, I saw pregnant women on every block. Strollers veered across my path, threatening to push me off the sidewalk and into the oncoming traffic. My rational side said I was being overly sensitive, but my irrational side wanted any woman who had ovulated in the past twenty-four hours banned from the neighborhood. Not too much to ask, right?

And I'm not alone. A good friend of mine who was also facing infertility called one day to tell me she had experienced the "holy trinity of babymaking" in a local CVS pharmacy: leafing through a magazine while she waited for her prescription, she came upon an article about Celine Dion and her IVF baby. As she read, she was distracted by a conversation between a very pregnant woman and the pharmacist. The woman was telling him how unprepared she felt for the baby. She was thrilled to be having it, but it "wasn't exactly planned." As my friend listened, page still open to Celine's drooling bundle of joy, another woman walked up to the counter with a child, who because of his race was obviously not genetically related to her. She asked if the pharmacist could recommend some kind of allergy medicine for "her son." God was clearly sending my friend a message.

"There it was, right in front of me," she said, "the three ways to have a baby. Get pregnant like a normal person, go high tech with IVF, or adopt." It all seemed so simple at the CVS.

The good news and the bad news for my husband and me was that we found out exactly what our problem was. We were diagnosed relatively quickly, after just a year of trying, unlike many couples who may never find out why they can't get pregnant naturally. In that respect we were lucky. My husband's issues showed up very clearly under the microscope. We knew he had sperm; they just needed some help. That's where I felt we were unlucky; I still wish it had been me.

Without making a gross generalization—okay, so it's a gross generalization—I believe that women handle infertility better than men do. I found this in our own experience as well as in my research. Statistics show that infertility affects men and women equally, but right from the start I assumed that *our* problem was *my* problem. I gave very little thought to the possibility that it could be my athletic, energetic, six-foot-four husband. I took full responsibility: I was too old, I'd been on the pill too long, I'd stood in front of too many satellite dishes, my job was too stressful, *I* was too stressful. Find a fault and it was mine.

The strange thing was that while I felt responsible for our infertility and hurt by my circumstances, I never really felt ashamed. I talked about it with my close friends and family, looking to find answers in their experiences, but when we found out it wasn't me, the bubble of silence descended. My husband told me, in no uncertain terms, to keep it quiet, and to know him is to know that's unlike him.

My husband, Scott, is one of the most outgoing, gregarious people I have ever known. He'll strike up a conversation with just about anybody on any topic. He and our FedEx guy are on a first-name basis. Infertility is the one exception. Even now, when most of our friends know we did IVF, we rarely tell them why.

Scott has always been a hard worker, like me, but for different reasons. As a very young boy, doctors told his parents that he was "slow." He wasn't retarded, they said, but he would never learn to ride a bicycle, never go to college, never be a great thinker. Never happened.

Scott rides a bicycle just fine, but nobody taught him how. His parents never pushed him, but they didn't treat him much differently than a normal child either. He had training wheels on his first bike, and one day, they simply fell off. Nobody noticed, and he kept on riding.

That's how most things happen for him, effortlessly. By the sixth grade, someone figured out that Scott wasn't slow, he was dyslexic, and with a little extra help, he was just as capable as any other kid in his class. He graduated high school and college and is the only person I know who actually read De Tocqueville's *Democracy in America* cover to cover. He is insatiably curious and marvelously bright, but infertility, unlike a learning disability, was not something he could just work harder at to fix. We both had the same problem, but it affected us in different ways.

Infertility seems to strike deeper into a man's character than it does a woman's. They often assume it means they are less strong, less virile, less masculine. I know of one man who refused to tell anyone of his problem, even his parents. He was so completely ashamed that he would interrogate his wife every week to make sure she hadn't told any of her friends or family. He quickly jumped to the conclusion that God didn't want him to reproduce, that he was unworthy. He had a hard time even thinking about adoption or artificial insemination because he felt his medical condition was a sign that he was not meant to be a parent; he simply wasn't a good enough person to raise a child. And he adored children.

Of the couples who declined to be interviewed for this book, most had male-factor infertility. Women seem to want to discuss the issue and hear all the stories; men go to all lengths to hide it.

Scott was very proactive medically, reading everything he could find on the subject, but I quickly noticed changes in him after the diagnosis. He seemed suddenly a little less confident in general and a lot less interested in sex. As a small-business owner, an expert in brand marketing, his easy ability to network and schmooze has always impressed me; suddenly he seemed less aggressive. And he was always very close with his family, but it took him some time to break the news. When he finally did, he learned that his father had a similar problem, so it was likely genetic. Scott had always known that it took many years for his parents to conceive him, but the family folklore was always that his mother had an "irregular cycle." I still wish we had known that earlier.

Our experience with infertility, though not exactly quick and painless, was relatively short-lived. We were diagnosed in March and pregnant by September. For others the road can be a lot longer, whether by circumstance or by choice, and every couple will face infertility with a different understanding, ideology, and attitude.

In the course of my research, I saw infertility from more perspectives than I ever imagined, but in the end, I couldn't write about them all. Instead I chose five couples, whom you will get to know through their own words in the following pages. They come from different social, economic, and ideological backgrounds, and they all reacted to infertility differently. Their common bond is that in the end they all chose to try in vitro fertilization, and their reasons were all the same: it was their last chance to have a child, the last judgment by God or nature or whatever as to whether or not they would procreate; it was the court of last resort.

ALEXANDRA AND PETER

Peter proposed to Alexandra on the threshold, the threshold of the bathroom of their basement apartment in Georgetown. It was two days before Thanksgiving, Alexandra's favorite holiday, and her family was already in DC for the festivities. She was standing at the sink, putting cuticle oil on her fingers. He was standing outside the door, carrying long-stemmed roses. It wasn't exactly what Alexandra had imagined when she dreamed of this moment as a young girl. The ring, yes, the roses, definitely, but she expected to be standing by the ocean or atop the Eiffel Tower, not by the shower curtain. Still, it was right. She said yes, and he slipped a diamond ring onto her oily finger.

Later that evening, in their self-described moony state, Peter said, "And we're gonna have kids." Just like that. Alexandra says it was "shocking." She had always imagined she would have a family, but it was just so strange when that fantasy suddenly moved into the realm of reality.

Peter and Alexandra met as regional wire service reporters on Capitol Hill. They were both in their late twenties. She grew up in the affluence of New York's Upper East Side; he grew up a traveler. Peter was willing to try anything and even spent time in the Peace Corps. For the first two years of their marriage, they lived a free and easy life. They traveled whenever they liked, wherever they liked, and pursued their careers with abandon. After four years, they decided it was time to settle down and start the family they had often talked about. Alexandra was ready, but like her experience with the engagement itself, the process of getting pregnant wasn't quite as she'd imagined it would be.

PETER: Alexandra wasn't patient enough about the whole thing.

ALEXANDRA: Well, as you know, when you want to start, you want it to happen yesterday. We tried in August and September, and I happened to have an ob/gyn visit in October . . . I went and I was like, "I am trying to get pregnant, I am on a mission, what the hell is going on, what do I do?" She told me to calm down and have sex every other night.

The scientific definition of infertility is the inability to conceive a child after one full year of trying. Most doctors stick to that and don't want to entertain the possibility of a problem until that year is exhausted. Like me, however, Alexandra wasn't willing to wait that long. Her mother had had trouble conceiving her, and she didn't want to waste any time finding out if she too had a problem.

Peter, on the other hand, was willing to take more time. He is one of five siblings, so infertility didn't really factor into his mind-set. He is also extremely patient, unlike his wife. Alexandra describes him as the type of guy who can build or fix anything, because, unlike most men, he actually reads instructions. He has the patience to work through lengthy explanations, follow directions carefully and slowly, and persistently achieve his goals. Unfortunately that didn't translate into IVF. He didn't want to read up on infertility or look into the options. Alexandra found herself taking most of the initiative.

ALEXANDRA: I didn't ask for any tests. I think she might have said the thing about the year, but maybe not. I was just assuming it was going to happen like the next month. Then no October, no November, no December, and I got an appointment in the first week of January to see her again. I was like, "There is a problem." And she said, "There is not a problem, it hasn't even been six months."

Alexandra told her that her mother had had problems, but the doctor was not concerned about that.

"If you told me your sister had problems, then I would be concerned." Then she said you have to try for a year and she told me the whole growth curve about, you know, at the end of the year 80 percent of couples, blah, blah, and I said that's nice, and I said I want to see a specialist and she said my job is to keep you calm, and I said I would be calm when a specialist tells me to be calm. I was just very frustrated.

PETER: I understood it, I mean, I thought it was pretty rational to wait and let things work themselves out.

ALEXANDRA: And I did too, and I thought, actually I am just being impatient. But I wanted it so badly and I knew it couldn't hurt to see a fertility specialist. I wanted the specialist to tell me: we checked you out, there are no blockages, your husband's sperm is fine, go on your way. I just wanted to be tested. [The doctor] recommended three specialists. I remember feeling so strange about even calling them. I secretly stayed home from work one morning and made the phone calls.

It wasn't long before Alexandra found out she had an ovulatory disorder that was affecting her fertility. Because she was so aggressive in seeking out help early, she saved several more months of trying uselessly. Most doctors do tell couples to wait a year simply because it takes the average absolutely healthy couple six months to conceive a child. Doctors don't want couples jumping into fertility treatment unnecessarily, so they generally recommend a year. And that's fine for some, but frankly I think a year is an awfully long time to wait, peeing on ovulation predictors and building up your hopes every twenty-eight or so days, especially when you aren't in your twenties anymore. If you've been trying for six months, and you have the means to get some very basic tests, why not? It's only hurting your bank account, and if there actually is something wrong, better to know sooner than later.

ANNE AND MICHAEL

Anne and Michael are together today because a long time ago someone else was late. Anne was supposed to be set up with Larry. They had a date to meet with a small gathering of friends, but Larry was late. His best friend, Michael, was right on time, and by the time Larry showed up, Michael had left with Anne. Three days later Anne and Michael were essentially living together. Six months later they bought a house together. Two years later, they were married. Larry was the best man.

Anne and Michael describe each other as incompatible on paper. He grew up in a small town in Washington state, she was raised in New York City. He is Christian, she is Jewish. He is mellow, easygoing, relaxed. She is a drama queen, "totally intense," she says. But they both studied political science and ended up in Washington, DC, looking to get into politics. As the saying goes, opposites attract, and they definitely did.

Still, as easy as their relationship was, Anne always knew that a family would take much more work.

ANNE: Before we got married, I told him I was going to have problems conceiving. I had had irregular periods and no periods and stuff since I was a teenager. I just knew I was not going to have an easy time of it. I didn't have anything specifically wrong. I told him before we got married that I might not be able to have natural children and we might have to do extraordinary measures, so he was aware of that . . . we went into it knowing. I told him, but he didn't believe me.

MICHAEL: In the absence of any data, no real data points . . . I didn't take it really seriously.

Each had strong attitudes toward infertility. When I asked Anne what defines their relationship, she immediately answered: these attitudes. Their approach to infertility sums up the differences between them. He had unshakable faith, right from the start. She was ready to adopt before they even tried. I found this common in most of the couples I interviewed, probably because women take on the responsibility not just for being pregnant but for getting pregnant. Because pregnancy is essentially their operation from the start, they carry much more of the stress of success and failure. Both Anne and Michael wanted children very much, even though neither are particularly close with their families. They began talking about it very early on, even before they were married. Ironically, the subject came up in the context of birth control. Anne had never really used birth control because, even without medical evidence, she was sure she couldn't get pregnant. Michael insisted she go on the pill. Even though Anne is pro-choice, she had told him she could never have an abortion, and at that point, before they were married, Michael wasn't ready to be a father, so he wasn't taking any chances. Anne went on the pill.

Why was Anne so sure she was infertile? Fifteen years of unprotected sex, for one thing. She also had irregular periods and a family history of problems. Because of that, Anne seemed almost resigned to it. She didn't even seem particularly bothered by it, as many women would be. She sounded as if she had always planned to adopt. Michael, on the other hand, was almost as convinced as she was—in the other direction. He just didn't buy her attitude.

To this day, Anne and Michael's infertility is unexplained. Michael tested normal and although Anne's irregular menstrual cycle convinced her she couldn't conceive, she did produce eggs and doctors told her there was really no reason she shouldn't be able to get pregnant naturally. That was when her attitude changed. The intense side of her kicked in, and when, after six months of trying, they came up empty Anne decided to be proactive, intensely proactive. Suddenly their roles were reversed, and their troubles began.

Anne and Michael were both young, well-educated urban intellectuals with similar goals and a strong marital bond, but once infertility showed up it moved in right between them. Anne took her usual approach; she wanted to know everything. Michael, who was always the driving force behind having a natural child, seemed to expect it just to come to him; all he wanted to know was when and where he needed to show up.

ANNE: He was always very confident it would happen. I came home one day, and I think I threw a fertility book at him and said, "I'm done. You don't seem to care. You don't come to appointments with me. I've given you fertility books, you don't read them, you have no idea what's going on, I'm shooting myself up with drugs over here and you don't know what they are, you don't seem to care, and I'm like, the hell with you! You want a natural child, go find someone else to have one!" And I wasn't even pissed. I was but I was more, I don't want this that badly. I'm okay without doing this, so if this is not that important to you that you're not going to get that involved, fine. We had three years to talk about how we would raise children, and I'd said from the beginning, "I want a partner. I want a full partner." When I threw the book at him, I was like, if this is any indication about how you're going to be as a parent, forget it! I don't want to do this! MICHAEL: She was right. It was a necessary turning point for the whole experience because it really did force the issue and got me very much more involved. I don't know if in the last however many months if I missed any of her appointments.

Michael needed to be hit over the head with it, literally, while Anne was going from doctor to doctor, getting herself tested and trying fertility drugs to make her ovulate more often. She wanted to try all the procedures she could, all the drugs and all the tests, everything except in vitro. Anne thought she knew all about IVF. She had read all the literature, but she was terrified of the procedure and swore she would never do it. If IVF was the only option left, she thought, then there were no more options. It would simply be time to adopt. Of this, she was certain, so she tried just about everything else.

ANNE: The doctor did the dye test. [This test involves shooting dye up the woman's fallopian tubes to find out if they are blocked.] He didn't mention that it was going to be so painful I could barely walk afterwards, and I went by myself. It was a horrible experience. I cramped terribly and it was terrible and my tubes were clear. I had heard anecdotal stories that sometimes women got pregnant after that test, because it kind of flushed you out. So we were kind of hopeful. I think I did the dye test before the [fertility drug] Clomid, but he put me on Clomid, and I had two cycles of just Clomid, and I got a breast lump. That was exciting. So I had to have surgery to have that removed.

Little by little Anne was running out of options. Adoption always lingered in the back of her mind. Michael wasn't prepared to give in. As is often the situation with such an emotional issue as infertility, firm plans and definite decisions began to waiver.

MICHAEL: It came up periodically. We had set some tentative timelines about how far we would go. We had left open at the beginning the question of the IVF. I'm the last male in my family, and so I was certainly more interested in having a natural child than adopting, at least initially.

ANNE: I was more interested in adopting. I would have adopted from the beginning and not gone through this.

MICHAEL: We wanted to make sure that while it was an important piece of our life, we weren't going to allow it to completely control our life, so, if it turned out that we were scheduled to be on vacation or something at a time when it was clear that we were supposed to be at the fertility clinic, we just made the decision that we would just skip that month.

ANNE: I was thirty when we started. That's one of the reasons we weren't driven to the every-month thing.

MICHAEL: But we'd talked it through and were also cognizant that sometimes you talk through the great plan and you get to the second stage of a plan, and everything changes in front of you. So we had that talk, and then we had another talk, and then a subsequent talk, and so on and so forth.

ANNE: Pressure is the wrong word. I knew it was his preference. I felt that I would go as far as I could to try to achieve that, to try to . . . achieve a natural birth. I was just mostly scared of the whole process. They almost couldn't do the breast surgery because I was so hysterical that I wouldn't let anybody . . . I mean it was bad. I went to see a phobia specialist because I was so just over-the-top scared. It's not rational what you're afraid of, and I was fairly adamant in the beginning. I wouldn't do IVF. You know . . . and then things change. Three and a half years later.

Three and a half years later, with all of the other options exhausted, Anne was ready to try IVF. She had been through so much already that after awhile the fear of IVF began to lessen. After all, she had been taking shots, she had had surgery, and IVF wasn't much more than that, right? Michael's desire to have a biological child was still strong, and Anne's desire to give him one was still strong enough.

TIM AND KATHY

Tim and Kathy have always considered themselves lucky. Even when it seemed like things weren't going their way, whatever it was that they wanted somehow found them. All they had to do was kiss the Blarney Stone, literally.

They were a lot alike. Both were raised in large, close-knit Catholic families. Both were interested in broadcast news. Both had attended Emerson College in Boston at the same time, but they first met several years later at an alumni dinner in Washington. They sat across from each other at the dinner table, and by the time the entrée was served, Tim knew this was the girl he was going to marry. Since Tim was living in DC and Kathy was in Boston, they wrote back and forth for a time. Soon Tim quit his job at a radio station to be with his love. Unfortunately, the job market in Boston was tight, so he was forced to work as a room-service waiter at a hotel. Not exactly his dream.

Then Kathy got a job at a television station in Vermont. They happened to have another position open, so she told the news director she knew a perfect guy for the job. She never told him it was her boyfriend. Fate landed them together again—and chipped in a bonus: Kathy won a balloon ride in a station raffle. There, a mile high, sailing into a warm pink sky, Tim proposed. She was holding a hot dog. He was holding his grandmother's diamond ring.

But Vermont wasn't exactly where either of them wanted to end up. That's when Tim went to Ireland and kissed the Blarney Stone. When he returned from his trip, there was a call from New England Cable News, the place he most wanted to work. They had a full-time job available. Tim calls himself a lucky guy, but the truth is he works hard to find his luck. By the time they were ready to get married, both had jobs in Boston, and everything was just as it should be. Then they tried to get pregnant.

Kathy's best friend, her maid of honor, had been battling infertility for years and had gone through no fewer than *seven* IVF cycles. Kathy was always there for her, on the end of the phone, at the doctor's office, in her living room, listening, consoling, and doing her best to help her friend through the disappointments. Kathy tried to give encouragement however she could, but *at the time* she herself couldn't exactly relate.

Kathy came from a large Catholic family in which it seemed like kids just grew on trees. Infertility never came up. It never had to. So as the years passed and her friend remained childless, Kathy just dished out the sympathy. She couldn't exactly put herself in her friend's shoes; who would want to? Then one day, Kathy looked down and realized she was wearing her friend's shoes.

KATHY: My mom had four kids, her mother had eight kids, so I figured I was at least good for two, you know? And Irish Catholic, I mean, come on? It's not until you do all the steps and have that test in the hospital where they blow out your tubes . . . telling work, I'll be in a little late . . .We didn't seek a specialist until we exhausted all other options. We just hoped it would evolve and it never did.

TIM: There's no good time to have a baby. It's never a perfect opportunity, so we were waiting to get a little more secure in our work and just to try to have things in a little better situation, and then when we were really really ready to have kids, all of a sudden, uh-oh, it's not working!

When they first started trying to get pregnant, Tim and Kathy both worked at a large local television station in Boston; he as a cameraman, and she as a producer. To them, everything was (and still is) a story, and they had each heard plenty of stories about couples struggling with infertility. Tim had done news pieces on extraordinary advances in infertility treatment, taping interviews with top specialists and their patients. Tim and Kathy were young, healthy, and active, and both came from families that had no history of infertility. At first, they decided that the only reason they weren't pregnant was because they weren't trying enough. Kathy now regrets that attitude. She regrets that she hesitated to get serious opinions; she regrets that she wasted four years of her life not giving it her all.

> KATHY: I wasn't pushing it, you know what I mean, I wasn't pushing it because I never thought it would be my problem. I thought it would come eventually, and then when you get so wrapped up with your work and everything, you don't really realize how much time is going by. At the same time we were going through it, my best friend was going through it. I never thought it would be me too.

After four years, though, they finally admitted they had a problem and decided to attack. Because of their experiences, they approached their problem with similar, almost businesslike attitudes, both expecting that no matter what, they would get pregnant eventually. They were equally committed. It was almost as if a light suddenly went on, and everything in their life became about the quest for a baby. For the first time in a long time, careers took a backseat.

Each went through a battery of tests. First it looked like Tim might have a low sperm count, but later tests showed he was fine. As for Kathy, she had one semiblocked fallopian tube, but her doctor said that should not affect her ability to get pregnant. To this day, Tim and Kathy's infertility is unexplained, which is surprisingly common. Many couples go through test after test and can't get a straight answer as to what's wrong.

KATHY: It would have been nice for him to have the problem and I could be like, "I'm fine!"—better psychologically for me. When we first thought it was his problem, I thought, "Great!" Not great, but you know.

Kathy says she most admires Tim because there is nothing he wouldn't do for her. Early on, someone once mentioned to her that Tim was the kind of guy who was so nice that no one would ever really appreciate him. Kathy did. She loved the fact that he was so devoted, not just to her, but to everything he did. Even though he often seemed lucky, she recognized that he worked hard to make his luck. IVF would be no different. Tim's only wish was that he could do all the work.

TIM: I could've carried a problem if it was mine a lot easier than hers because I can't help her, I can't fix it, I can't change it, I can just watch. That drives me crazy, when there's things like that that I can't fix.

CAROL AND MIKE

On the surface, Carol and Mike had little in common She was classical; he was rock 'n' roll. Carol was one of three daughters of a local Protestant minister. Mike was an army brat, the only child of a divorced father who took him to live in Japan, France, and Germany. Mike is ten years older than Carol. When they met, at a church, each was equally unimpressed.

Carol was applying for a job as the church organist. Mike was having lunch with the minister. It wasn't until a mutual friend begged him to take her out, that they finally shared a cup of coffee. Within a year, they decided to share their lives.

Both Carol and Mike were committed to family and wanted to have children, but they put it off a few years, while Carol went to graduate school in music. Mike pursued a career in tax law and accounting, and the two settled down to a quiet existence in Virginia.

About six years after they were married, Mike and Carol first started trying to conceive. It was 1985. Mike was more than forty years old at the time, so after a year without success, they decided to have him tested. The process to test him seemed less invasive than the tests for Carol. They didn't have a lot of money, and their insurance wasn't much help, but they figured the cost was worth it.

Mike's semen analysis shocked them both to the core. It showed him to be completely sterile, no sperm at all. After another few tests, they found the cause. His epididymis was completely blocked. The epididymis is the tube that the sperm normally runs through. The reason for the blockage was far more difficult to accept than most. It was the result of a massive previous injury.

MIKE: I was Special Forces during the Vietnam War. I was in Laos. I was captured, and I was beaten severely. That was the scarring.

The scarring was so bad that it had completely blocked the path for any sperm to get through. Mike survived being a prisoner of war, but his captors took away his ability to have children. After all he had been through and all he had gotten past emotionally, this was like being beaten all over again.

But Mike wasn't the type to give up all that easily. At the time, he read an article about a doctor in St. Louis who had run experiments in extracting epididymal sperm. Through an intricate operation, he could take the sperm out before it had to make its way through the tubes. Unfortunately, the science was not yet advanced enough to try, and his doctor told him it was at least five years away from being a viable alternative. He did, however, send him to a specialist to see if the epididymis could be cleared.

> MIKE: At that point we were so willing to try stuff. I had two surgeries to try to clear up the blockage. I felt like we should just put a zipper in there.

Neither surgery was a success, so at that point Carol and Mike were faced with a wrenching decision.

> MIKE: Carol had some problems with adoption. She'd known some families who adopted kids that didn't turn out terribly well . . . that was when we went through the rather agonizing decision to use donor sperm or not. We decided yes, we would be better off having a child that was biologically related to one of us.

Mike had no choice but to give up on his own dreams of ever being a biological father. He went through a period of grieving and then decided that he shouldn't deprive Carol of the experience of having her own child.

> MIKE: The comment was made one evening, "I haven't gone through however many years it was of having

periods, to not have a kid!" She never knew what she was getting into.

They never knew what *they* were getting into—a decade-long roller-coaster ride. They began by using donor sperm. Carol had no reason to believe there was anything wrong with her, so she expected to get pregnant quite easily. The infertility was his issue after all. She tried several times, but over and over again it just didn't seem to work. It would be a cruel coincidence to find out they both had a problem.

Then Carol tried going on the fertility drug Clomid and went through several invasive tests, but doctors could find nothing wrong. The bad news was, this added more years of frustration. Still, they weren't ready to jump to IVF.

CAROL: The cost was quite a lot more at that point and that was getting to the time frame when taking sperm from Michael was on the horizon. We just sort of didn't do anything for a while.

MIKE: We were relying a lot on the doctors for advice. We said okay, where do we go from here?

Looking back, Mike now feels that the fertility specialist cost them valuable time. The clinic they were using didn't perform IVF and recommending the procedure would have meant losing a patient; Mike felt that was why the doctor kept telling them to use the donor sperm with the Clomid.

Ironically, they spent so long going through testing and drug therapies that by the time they had reached the end of that rope, technology had advanced and suddenly Mike had a new option. That doctor in St. Louis, the one who was extracting epididymal sperm, was ready to take him—for $20,000.

CAROL: It was a chance!
MIKE: This was the chance to have our kid. I flew to St. Louis, and I had it done. I stayed in St. Louis for the next day. I was not allowed to walk. I had to get a wheelchair to the airport. They came with the wheelchair at the airplane, and I had to be in bed for I think three days after that.

The surgeon said my operation was the most difficult he'd ever seen, the worst scarring he'd ever seen, but in the process of doing the surgery, he did withdraw some epididymal sperm, which he tested, and it was viable and all that, so we froze it.
CAROL: Three vials! There were three or four vials of sperm that he took during that surgery.

The only way to use the sperm was through in vitro fertilization because (without getting too medical) of the nature of epididymal sperm—it doesn't really swim—which necessitates injecting it into the egg. IVF would give Mike a second chance at being a natural father. The natural gift that had been taken away so brutally, he thought, was being returned to him through the magic of modern science.

CHRIS AND KATE

The night Chris met Kate, he wrote his phone number on an enormous male blow-up doll. All the guys were doing it. Kate was at a bachelorette party for her cousin at a bar in Orlando, Florida. Chris, who was training to be a fireman, just happened to be at the same bar with a police officer friend of his. It only took a few minutes of talking to Kate, and Chris knew he'd better get his name on that doll.

> CHRIS: I thought all the good ones were already married. I wasn't having a whole lot of luck being the single guy. I really thought it was too good to be true. This isn't going to work out as I hoped. And if she would have known all those expectations that night, I'm sure I would have scared her right out of the room.

But what kind of expectations can a girl have of a guy who writes his phone number on a blow-up doll that just so happens to be handcuffed to her not-so-sober cousin? Apparently, great expectations. Chris wasn't stupid; he made sure he got Kate's number too, and he called her the moment he got home and left a message to let her know he wasn't just some guy in a bar.

An avid photographer, Chris had gone to work in the profession but quickly found the business side sucking out all his creative energies. Always on the road, shooting at different locations, it didn't take long for him to realize that this was not his calling. He wanted roots. He wanted a family. He wanted out.

Then tragedy opened a new door. Chris was very close to an uncle who was about his age. The uncle adored motorcycles, fast motorcycles, and one night his life came crashing to an end on a dark road in Albany, New York. Chris traveled to the funeral from Florida and found himself at the scene of the crash just one day later. The road was still scattered with the litter of lifesaving equipment.

Emergency medical service supplies, plastic bags, sterile wrappers, a rubber glove. Someone had come to this spot on this road to save a life, Chris thought. That someone had a real purpose. Chris felt he had no purpose. Suddenly he did. Chris's uncle was a firefighter. He would continue his uncle's work.

Kate got the same inspiration from her mother. Not a tragic story, thankfully, as her mother is still alive and well. Kate's mother is a teacher, and growing up, Kate felt there was simply no more rewarding profession on earth. She thought about being a nurse, but she didn't like giving people shots. Teaching was it. She adored children, especially the little ones.

So the teacher and the fireman met in a bar, and the teacher and the fireman fell in love. Chris knew within the first month that this was the girl he wanted to marry, but he figured he'd better wait an acceptable period of time before he asked.

They were married in July and by October began trying to have a child. Kate, who was twenty-nine at the time, had a thyroid problem, but her doctor assured her he could get it under control and it should have no effect on her fertility.

CHRIS: We both automatically just saw ourselves as parents.
KATE: I was hoping it would happen in six to nine months. I had that in my head. At nine months I started to worry and wonder why. I had always had this feeling that I wouldn't be able to get pregnant. I went to the doctor for my yearly and I told her we had been trying and that nothing was happening. She said, "You shouldn't worry, you haven't been trying for a year yet. Why don't you just have some wine and try again, and you might get pregnant." Really, that's what she

said to me, and I said, "Well when are you going to do some tests to tell me everything's okay?" She said I had to wait until we had been trying for a year.

I was very upset because I felt that I knew my body and I felt that there was something wrong, and me getting drunk and having sex was not going to get me pregnant, and I wanted her to do something about it.

CHRIS: I checked out fairly early in the process. I had a lot of denial going, and I said, okay, you know it's not working, it just takes time. I just thought we were anxious and eager.

KATE: My doctor ordered an ultrasound. She told me I had a cyst, and it turned out not to be a cyst. That was probably at a year.

Then they did a test, the dye test, and that's when they referred us to an infertility specialist. One of my tubes was blocked and infected. I was so unhappy at the doctor's office. They were mean and rude and didn't call me with the results of tests, and finally a doctor in the practice, not my doctor, called us in and told me it was blocked and then referred me to another infertility specialist for a laparoscopy.

CHRIS: We had friends who had gone through this. Our neighbors across the street were going through the same problems and were doing IVF and knew this doctor.

KATE: They went in and found that my left fallopian tube was very infected and had all this nasty fluid in it. He told us going in that he would be able to check out the other things and if it was good he would keep it in but if it was bad he would have to take it out. So they went in and he found that the tube was really infected, and he had to remove it.

He left the right tube, which he said wasn't in great condition, but he thought that we would be able, with some help, to get pregnant.

Kate and Chris, like so many others, started with a less invasive fertility method, using some drugs to make Kate produce more eggs and using artificial insemination with Chris's sperm (I'll explain this procedure in more detail later). Within a few months, it worked.

KATE: I got pregnant with an insemination in June 2001. This was a year after my surgery. I couldn't believe that I actually was pregnant, but I was, but then things kept getting worse. The doctor told me to come back at seven weeks and we'll listen to the heartbeat. Every day I just, I just . . . couldn't wait for the day to get over and I was so worried because I just wanted to be okay. Oh it was so hard.

CHRIS: I was very optimistic at that point. I still was thinking, maybe a little denial, but I was just thinking, hey, we're there.

KATE: I didn't want to tell anybody, and I remember my sister calling me and asking me, and I didn't want to tell her. I told my mother, but I said I didn't want anybody to know because what if something bad happens. And she said, "Well wouldn't you want your family to know and to be able to be there for you in case it doesn't happen?" So I told my sisters, and they were so excited.

But the excitement wouldn't last long.

KATE: First I was spotting, then I was in all this pain. I would go in there . . . to do my blood and they were like, "No no no, you're fine. Your levels are climbing, everything's okay. It's not ectopic." They had told me that I might have an ectopic pregnancy, so that was always in my head and then I would come home and everything's safe, well then I kept bleeding and then I was in pain, and I kept telling them I know something's wrong, I know something's wrong, and then I go in two days before they're supposed to be looking for a heartbeat and he does an ultrasound and has to tell us that the sac is not in the uterus, it's someplace else, and I'm so sorry but it's not a healthy pregnancy. At least we had the nice doctor to tell us that.

My body was miscarrying and getting rid of it on its own.

The risk of ectopic pregnancy was simply too much. Kate's body could not safely transport an embryo through her one remaining fallopian tube.

CHRIS: The doctor said stop.
KATE: What he said was, "Stop because ectopic is bad, you're lucky your body did what it needed to do. Don't do anything." So he did another test in August to see how my remaining tube was and when he did that one, that's when he really said, "It's not good, I want you to stop trying to get pregnant."
CHRIS: He used some language that was descriptive. At the time I had some familiarization with ectopic pregnancies,

and he said, you know it could kill Kate, if it were to rupture or something like that. He said we still have alternatives at this point, don't try to get pregnant right now. We had one ectopic pregnancy, and there's a very high likelihood that the same thing would happen again, and we might not have the same results where her body took care of things on its own.

He was so ultra-concerned that I was adamant, no way. My desire to have children was never ever, never once greater than my desire to keep Kate around.

An ectopic pregnancy occurs when the embryo lodges itself in the fallopian tube and doesn't settle in the uterus where it should. IVF is a perfect solution for those who are prone to ectopic pregnancies or who have blocked or missing fallopian tubes. That's because IVF completely bypasses the tubes. The eggs are retrieved from the ovaries, fertilized in a laboratory dish, and then deposited directly into the uterus. If you have trouble with your tubes, there's really no other way to get pregnant.

And that's where Chris and Kate and so many others end up, with no choice. Infertility can have many causes, but there are really very few remedies. Surgery can cure blockage, male or female, and fertility drugs can help a woman to produce more eggs, giving the couple better odds. Most of us will try the various, easier, cheaper, less invasive methods, and, depending on our unique character as a couple, we will devote X number of years to trying. But when all else fails, there is only one last chance, one last choice, and one final question: do we go high tech?

CHAPTER 2

TAKING THE LEAP

I can't say I ever expected to get as far as in vitro fertilization. I always assumed something else would work. That something else was "turkey basting," and that would definitely be the answer, since our infertility was male factor. Turkey basting is the adorable buzzphrase used to describe my monthly rendezvous with a catheter. The scientific term is intrauterine insemination (IUI). I was convinced it would work. It simply had to.

How did it work? Every month, when my little computerized fertility monitor (only $200 from CVS.com) blinked that I was about to ovulate, my husband and I would have an exceptionally romantic morning. He would get up at 6 A.M. and head for the fertility specialist's office. There, he would be sent to a little room with a few erotic magazines and ejaculate into a cup. From 7 A.M to 10 A.M, lab technicians somewhere in the same building would "wash" his sperm, removing the dead or slow ones and leaving us with a "clean" specimen of less voluminous but more viable sperm. By 10 A.M, I would arrive at the same little office. Using a catheter, the doctor would then shoot this sample past my cervix and hopefully as close to my emerging egg as possible. Something like basting a turkey inside, but a lot less romantic.

This is how we spent a summer. We did it three times, and three times it didn't work. Most of the couples I spoke to tried this method, with and without fertility drugs, several times. One couple I know has tried it about eight times because the woman is so afraid to do IVF. IUI has pretty much replaced sex in their lives.

Even though the success rates for IUI are much lower than they are for IVF, the procedure somehow seems more natural and easier to accept, and that's why most of us do it first. Plus, it only costs about $300 a hit, compared with up to $12,000 for IVF. It's hard to know the success rates for IUI because it is not required by law to be tracked like IVF.

After our third try, the doctor came back with some bad news. It seemed that each month Scott's count and motility (ability of sperm to swim) were getting worse and worse. He told us very matter-of-factly that we could keep trying this, and maybe it would work. He also told us that given our problem, we could eventually get pregnant on our own, but it would probably take many many years, and there were no guarantees. Then he said, "If you want to get pregnant now, we need to be more aggressive." Aggressive meant IVF.

For us, the choice was not as difficult as it was for others. I certainly had fears, most of which revolved around the question of would an IVF baby be "normal"? I knew that the procedure had been around for twenty years, but I still wondered if there were some hidden abnormalities that just hadn't surfaced yet. Would the baby look different? Would it be retarded in some way? Would it have emotional difficulties?

Another concern was the type of IVF we were going to try: ICSI (intracytoplasmic sperm injection). ICSI is the advanced form of IVF that came into practice about a decade ago. Instead of putting the sperm and egg in a dish and hoping they'll get together, the technicians take one sperm into a tiny needle and actually inject it directly into the egg. In natural fertilization, only part of the sperm gets into the egg because the sperm sheds its tail in the process. In ICSI, the entire body of the sperm enters the egg. Since it hasn't been around all that long, no one knows if this type of fertilization has any direct effect on the later development of a child, but major IVF centers in the biggest U.S. cities are using this procedure far more often than traditional IVF. It just works better.

As a journalist, though, I always fear the scam. I had read the statistics on ICSI, and it occurred to me that perhaps all these clinics weren't being as careful as they should be, that they were doing ICSI not because it was such a wonderful new improvement, but because it would up their success rates and make them look better in the increasingly competitive fertility market. Maybe this procedure wasn't really ready for use on humans. This could be a huge story, I thought. I could hear the TV news anchor's lead in my head now, or, ten years from now: "In the news tonight, thousands of adolescents in America are growing a third arm, the result of big-money baby scams. Fertility doctors hid the secret for more than a decade. Quick-fix ICSI! Is your child at risk?"

This is the kind of ridiculousness that runs through your head in the middle of the night, as you ponder the possibility of trusting the creation of your child to some guy in a laboratory whom you'll probably never meet, instead of to God or to fate or whatever particular stork you happen to believe in. I just didn't know what to think. I knew ICSI was being done, and I knew that it was our best chance for success, but I worried. I didn't tell my husband how much I worried about that; I was just a little too ashamed because all I should have been worried about was would it work.

I can't say I was worried about the actual procedure though. I've never been seriously ill a day in my life, and I have always been pretty good about giving blood and getting shots. I was still young enough to feel physically invincible, and since the infertility was not my issue, I felt it would work.

Scott was more concerned about my having to go through all the shots and drugs. He also felt very guilty that it was his problem, and yet I had to do all the work. But the bottom line was that all these fears and all the guilt were nothing compared to our equally desperate desire to have a child. I don't even think we discussed it very much. It was just our only option, the last resort.

Alexandra and Peter felt the same way, but for them fear was not a factor. They weren't doing ICSI, and they had a very strong belief in the science as a whole. They also felt that because they were young and still within the normal age range for having children, that they weren't doing anything outlandish. They both had this very strong conviction that they deserved to have a child, and nothing was going to stand in their way.

PETER: . . . just because there's a quarter-century track record. All things are relative. If you've got an ethical problem with that process, that's one thing. I consider myself a very practical person. Taking things too far is when you are pushing things beyond what is reasonably possible and this is clearly reasonably possible, and probable even.

ALEXANDRA: I consider myself a spiritual person on some level. Peter is a reformed Catholic—he's rejected it. I really felt different than some of those stories I've heard like of the woman who's forty-two and has done in vitro. To me that was like keeping the dead grandfather alive on the ventilator machine. That was so depressing to me I couldn't take it. But I felt that I was young and at the beginning of this in vitro road; I would try it and we could end up with our miracle and science was there for me; it was going to save my situation.

PETER: We are responsible folks who are educated and can give children a good life. It is a little manipulative for the human system, but it's all for a good end.

ALEXANDRA: I felt it was like a miracle, it was a miraculous discovery that they made, that they could do this, and I actually felt really positive about the whole thing; I don't have a problem with the fact that only the best [embryos] made it to the top. I felt like we were going to have these great embryos that were really tough stuff, and we did.

Alexandra was also tired of pumping herself full of drugs that weren't working.

ALEXANDRA: I just wasn't responding, I will never forget on the second one. They want you to make a few big ones [produce a lot of eggs in one cycle], and I was making a lot of medium size and a lot of small ones too. At the end when they get you to that trigger day, when they see you and they're like—it's coming around that time—you're like I guess we'll trigger you today [induce ovulation] and they were so disappointed and I thought, what the fuck . . . am I doing to myself, you know?

PETER: That was a big issue. Alexandra was always—every other day, she would comment on the drugs she was pumping into her body. Foreign substances are not necessarily going to manifest into something later, but she was just opposed to polluting her body with things that weren't already there. My impression was they were just extra hormones, but I really don't know what they are.

ALEXANDRA: Your hormone balance is like some God given natural thing and you're not supposed to throw it out of whack.

PETER: I thought it was better than a lot of things you can put into your body.

ALEXANDRA: At least in vitro is more precise.

That made their decision pretty simple, but for Anne and Michael, it took longer to come around. As I described earlier, Anne was petrified of the IVF procedure and far more inclined to adopt.

ANNE: We had these deals going on. I told him at first I would never do IVF because I had heard a long time ago that the retrieval was horribly painful. They used to do it with you awake. I had medical phobias and I didn't want to have surgery. I hated to have blood taken.

But after several years, procedures and even abdominal surgery, Anne was ready. After all, she'd been through so much already. To stop now, when there was one more possibility, a really good possibility, suddenly seemed unacceptable. Anne would stare down her fears and attack IVF the way she had all the other fertility procedures they had tried. She and Michael made one more agreement.

MICHAEL: At that point we had made the decision that we were going to try IVF. We had also decided that we were going to do this no more than three times. We were going to max out [at] three.

ANNE: I remember reading statistics that said after three times your chances went way down.

MICHAEL: We had agreed that if it was meant to be it was going to be and the idea of going through it over and over . . . I don't consider that to be medical so much as at some point you've got to say *no mas*. Who's to say that . . . lawn mower, pull three times and the third almost kicks, who's to say we wouldn't try a fourth, but at that point at least, our nineteenth final plan was that we were just going to do three IVFs.

ANNE: I was really excited about the IVF actually because I wanted to know . . . the only thing they hadn't looked at were my eggs, and so I figured . . . I wanted to know what my eggs looked like. That's the only way I'm going to find out. Maybe they were defective. I was excited, anxious to do it from that perspective. If all my eggs came up fours and fives [low quality on a one-to-five scale, one being the best] or didn't fertilize, we probably wouldn't have gone on at that point.

Carol and Mike didn't have the luxury of choices and options. Mike decided he wasn't going to go through the surgery again to have epididymal sperm extracted. They had only three vials of sperm, tucked away in the freezer, and they were going to be as aggressive as they could be when it came to using them. They could have done artificial insemination, but doctors told them it would likely be a waste of time and a waste of that valuable sperm. The best hope of fertilization was through IVF. Because it was epididymal sperm, which is not as mobile, they had to do ICSI. Again, they had no choice in the matter.

MIKE: They'd explained to us exactly what it was. They had nice little eight-by-ten glossy pictures, little drawings of this is . . . what they do.
CAROL: It was the only shot we had.

Like Alexandra and Peter, their only fear was that it wouldn't work. They didn't seem to worry about the science, as I did.

MIKE: Regular in vitro had been going on for a number of years at this point, and the [ICSI] kids were now grade school age, and by all reports were doing just fine.
CAROL: We were within the first couple of years of ICSI and we just said that is it.
MIKE: They came up with some pretty good stuff about the normal pregnancies and the kids. They really hadn't had any real incidence of birth defects or anything like that coming out of it, which I guess was the biggest concern. Hey, I trust science. I trusted doctors . . . at that point.

Tim and Kathy trusted the facts. Once again, they approached it as journalists and used their experiences as guideposts. Fear didn't factor into their decision at all. In fact, Tim didn't even consider that it might not work for them.

TIM: I'd done a few stories, I'd been exposed to this, talked to doctors, and I was convinced it works a hundred percent before we even started this, and I knew, watching Debby (Kathy's friend) go through it, it could take some time, it could be hard, but I know this works. There's no doubt in my mind, there was no second-guessing this, this is a silver bullet that is going to have results sooner or later. I felt like the sooner we started using this, the sooner we'd have the results we wanted.

And Kathy had had enough of trying other methods, like turkey basting. She thought a lot about doing IVF but didn't really jump on board until one of the nurses at her clinic made the decision for her.

KATHY: They would see the disappointment on my face and, you know, you would kind of get attached to nurses and certain people, and they're like, just go right for IVF, and so I said, I'm going to go right for that, because it wasn't an insurance thing, our insurance would pay. . . Some people go on Clomid and get pregnant, so we wanted to try at least, because maybe that would work, but when it didn't after two tries it's like, this is done.

It was a one-in-ten chance with IUI and with in vitro it was one in four, so the odds are much better. She just told me, forget this, and I did, I said okay, next time, go with my choice.

TIM: We did, in a lot of ways, choose the path of least resistance because we did have these options with the insurance, and we did have a doctor who also believed in that: "Let's go for the cure, let's not get hung up on what's wrong." You pick your battles, and we picked our battles pretty selectively, what we wanted to worry about, what we wanted to think about, how we wanted to feel. We really tried to talk it over and say, "All right, this is just a big hassle, it's just a science project."

The facts and statistics about IVF helped Tim and Kathy to overcome their fears, but they had another hurdle to face. Both are Catholic and both were well aware that the Catholic church frowns on in vitro.

TIM: We're extremely respectful of life and we have other decisions to make down the road.

KATHY: We always wanted to have a family and isn't that what marriage is about?

TIM: We want to raise our child as a Catholic, with the church, and I personally didn't see a real problem with it. I chose not to fight it; this is not my battle.

Kathy: I didn't want to make it a huge issue. Obviously we haven't come into a situation where it was an issue. They don't know.

TIM: Other religions are pretty clear about how life starts. Life starts inside the womb, not outside. I guess it could be convenient to adopt other religious beliefs, but we made our choice to go ahead with this, and we found it morally acceptable. I think that everybody we came in contact with in the medical profession was also morally respectful, morally proper in the handling of the whole issue. It seems like the church is in the middle of all these great questions now, and I don't think we sidestepped their opinion.

KATHY: We didn't broadcast it either.

TIM: We had to make a choice. It was either this or not have kids. We could have adopted, we could have gone down that road, which is just as complicated. It's pick your fight, and we chose this way, and I would gladly sit down with a priest and have a discussion with him about this. I never did. Maybe I probably should have, but I just felt that morally this was okay.

Both Tim and Kathy were lucky to have supportive families. That's not always the case. I know of another Catholic couple who conceived a child through IVF. The woman's parents were so appalled that they didn't speak to her for more than a year and missed seeing their grandchild as an infant. Others I've spoken to struggled hard with the moral issues of IVF. They felt that if God hadn't meant for them to have a child, then who were they to mess with nature? The answer to that, many found in the end, is if God didn't want couples to do IVF, it wouldn't exist as an option. That was Anne's opinion:

ANNE: I felt nervous because if God had intended for me to have children I would get pregnant, or maybe there was a baby out there who was meant to be adopted by us. But I felt pretty confident that if we got pregnant, then that was what was supposed to happen. So when you talk about manipulating nature, I'm a believer in fate. I use the word God, but for me, God made the medicine too. It's like saying, "I won't get on an airplane because I don't have wings." I don't see much difference between the two.

For Chris and Kate, again, there were no other options. Kate's doctor told her in no uncertain terms that if she tried to get pregnant using her one remaining fallopian tube, she would be risking an ectopic pregnancy that could ultimately kill her. Chris was willing to take risks fighting fires, but he was adamant about Kate's safety. He found himself in a tough situation.

CHRIS: I wanted a biological child so much. As the process wore on, I was adamant against adoption. I wouldn't even go there. I wouldn't even think about that sort of thing.

Neither Chris nor Kate was particularly afraid of the science either. In fact, they said they never even considered that it might be a risk.

KATE: The thought never crossed our minds.
CHRIS: The doctor put our minds at ease with regards to several things. I mean, first off, he said, "You know when you hear the stories about the five, eight, ten children, you know, that is not going to happen to you." In his opinion that was reckless. That's something you can control.

As for the relative newness of the science, they never really considered it, and I have to say that was one of the most surprising things I found in my research. Yes, IVF has been around for a quarter of a century, but, to me at least, it really only seems to have gone mainstream in the last five years or so. Maybe I'm wrong, maybe it just wasn't on my radar screen, so I didn't notice, but a lot of people I spoke with seemed surprised at this question: are you worried about the science itself? Most people answered: "Well we were worried that it wouldn't work." It was almost as if people didn't understand what I was talking about, as if doing IVF were like getting a nose job. To them, it was a choice, but not a risk. I still wonder about the science and probably will until my kids are grown and have their own kids.

My own fears were about the science of ICSI, which again is creating an embryo in a different way than it naturally occurs, by allowing the tail of the sperm to enter the mix. Recent studies in Australia have shown that there is absolutely no difference between a regular IVF child and an ICSI child, but since the science is still not that old, I had fears.

The questions that are now being asked more in the field are about the drug regimens used to produce all those extra eggs and to make the uterine environment acceptable for implantation. I'll address all of this later when we get to the actual procedure, but again, I was surprised at how few of the couples worried about the science itself.

The biggest issue I found was with religious couples. Chris and Kate weren't particularly religious at the time, although they, as many others, came to find comfort in religion more and more as the ordeal of infertility dragged on. For them, IVF was a last resort and therefore not so much a choice as a result.

For those who considered God in the equation, they seemed to take it from a practical stance. If God created the possibility of IVF, then what was so wrong with it? Obviously that argument has a million holes, since from that perspective you could say that God created any number of horrible things, like nuclear bombs and poison gas. But when I suggested that (carefully), most people said, "But look at the result!" Here is an option that is a wonder, a wonder of science. Like the polio vaccine or the future cure for cancer, this is the work of diligent scientists striving to help infertile couples realize a family.

One Catholic couple I spoke with had twin boys through in vitro fertilization. They named them Girard and Jude after the patron saint of infertility and the patron saint of lost causes.

CHAPTER 3

CHOOSING YOUR MAKER

According to the Centers for Disease Control, in 2001, 384 fertility clinics in the United States were vying for what has now become a multibillion dollar business. I called one of those clinics, a very popular shop in the DC metro area, which was recommended by that wonderful ob who fired me. The clinic had a fabulous Web site that advertised "The IVF Shared Risk Refund Plan: 100% refund unless you have a baby." It claimed this plan would offer "peace of mind during treatment." That's right, they offered a money-back guarantee if they couldn't get you pregnant in four tries of IVF—of course they couldn't give me an appointment for four months.

This is a prime example of what has come to be known as the IVF factory. It's one of the biggest complaints I found from many of the couples I spoke with. These clinics are so large and perform so many procedures on so many people that the service is not exactly personal.

An article in the *New York Times* on January 1, 2002, titled "Fertility Inc.: Clinics Race to Lure Clients" describes the "aggressive marketing" tactics of these clinics, which often employ their own marketing consultants. They offer wine-tasting dinners and entertainment for doctors to lure them into referrals. Then they advertise free counseling seminars for infertile couples in the hope that they'll choose their clinic as a result.

> *Infertility has become a big, fiercely competitive business, with a billion dollars in revenues and with more and more doctors fighting for a limited number of patients. The growth of the field has been fueled by rising success rates and increased demand from patients, many of whom pay tens of thousands of dollars out of their own pockets in hopes of having a child.*

In addition to that, fertility is actually the one medical specialty regulated by the government; thanks to the Fertility Clinic Success Rate and Certification Act of 1992, sponsored by Senator Ron Wyden of Oregon, clinics are actually required to report their success rates to the Centers for Disease Control. These statistics are then made available to the public in annual reports. On the plus side, it's easy to learn about the clinic you might be considering, but the downside is it creates greater competition. Clinics are increasingly sensitive about their success rates, and, therefore, as the article in the *New York Times* warns, some clinics end up performing "risky procedures," like implanting too many embryos, just to increase those rates, or they offer their money-back guarantees to "only the youngest and healthiest, who are most likely to get pregnant."

I considered going with the big clinic. I even made an appointment and read through its thick, glossy brochure, but in the end, I opted out and signed up with Preston Sacks, MD, a reproductive endocrinologist with a smaller practice and an enormous heart. He was recommended to us by a friend whose sister had used him with great success.

When I called Dr. Sacks's office to schedule an appointment for a consultation, the receptionist said he would give me a call back. Believe it or not, he did—*that afternoon!*—and we talked at length about our situation. When my husband and I went in to meet him, he spent more than an hour with us, drawing very inartful pictures of the human reproductive system but explaining away every question we could think of.

He also didn't pressure us to go straight to IVF. In fact, he didn't even suggest it. Many specialists will pressure their patients into IVF because it has a higher success rate than other methods and because it simply costs a whole lot more. It's their best moneymaker. Dr. Sacks recommended some tests for me first, just to make sure I was fine, and then suggested turkey basting.

It's rare to find a doctor with a really personal touch, but I found that in a situation as emotional as infertility, it is invaluable. Dr. Sacks was always on the other end of the phone or e-mail. He clearly loved his work—almost as much as he loved The Food Network. There I'd be, legs in the air, listening to him recount a recipe for vegetarian fois gras that he'd seen on *Emeril* the previous night, and before I knew it, whatever he was up to down there was over. He also approached the grueling testing phase with a great sense of humor. After I had the dye test, he greeted my husband by telling him this was "Blue Box Day." In other words, my husband had better get himself to Tiffany's fast for a little something shiny.

The bottom line is I trusted Dr. Sacks, and when you're faced with a science that doesn't often inspire trust, this is a crucial attribute. He talked us through everything, offered advice, and in the end left us to make our own decisions without pressure. He also didn't consider his job finished when he got us pregnant, but followed us through the pregnancy, offering invaluable guidance.

Choosing a specialist can be almost as hard as making the decision to do IVF. A friend of mine has now gone through several doctors. Unfortunately, few have inspired the kind of trust in her that Dr. Sacks did in me. She still has not made the decision to move to IVF, in part, I think, because she hasn't found the right specialist. If you don't trust the doctor, you can't trust the science.

Not everyone I spoke with had the same criteria for choosing a specialist. In fact, some wanted the factory, a facility that does thousands of IVF retrievals a year. The sheer volume of activity in such a place would reduce the fear factor, and a busy lab that is doing a billion procedures is presumably getting a lot of practice, doing it right more often than not. What a couple actually experiences during IVF is really a very small part of what is going on; many couples felt good to know that they had a big, well-funded, experienced lab processing their donations.

Alexandra and Peter went to a large facility but luckily sought out and found some very personal touches.

ALEXANDRA: I definitely felt like I was just on an assembly line, but my nurse and I ended up having a really good relationship. I knew she was talking to two dozen hysterical women every day like me . . . at first it was very hard because I would choke up on the phone with her. Eventually I started realizing that she was making all these accommodations, like after I would take the Clomid, five days later I would take the blood test to see if there was hormone surge at this proper time, and she would call me back on my cell phone and she would be patient if I was in a restaurant and it was loud and I would run into the street. This happened several times. And I began to think, wow, this woman is really trying to make me feel like I am the only one, much more the nurse than the doctor.

Tim and Kathy also went to a large facility because they wanted the quickest path to success. They didn't want to waste time with an exhaustive round of tests. They just wanted results and a doctor who could get them.

TIM: He said something like, "You want the car to run? Do you want to know what's wrong with it or do you want it to run? We can tear the car apart and find out what the problem is, or we can just get it going for you, and it would be a lot faster and probably easier just to get it going." That told me this is our man, this is our guy. He really had that mentality of let's do what's good for you, if you really need to know what's wrong with you, we'll do it, but if you want a baby, let's skip over this other stuff, so that's what we decided was the best thing to do. At first you're not under the clock and then all of a sudden you start feeling like, we might be under the clock!

KATHY: When we met him, we wanted the appointment so bad, and then you want it to go so fast, and it pretty much did go fast, for us.

Chris and Kate took a recommendation. Living in Florida, the old-age capital of the world, fertility clinics were not quite as numerous as in other areas of the country. Luckily, their neighbors had gone through IVF and recommended a specialist to them.

> KATE: In that practice there were three doctors, and when you first go, you can choose. The doctor that we saw we liked very, very much. He was very nice, very honest, you could trust him. I felt like, yes he's working for customers and making a lot of money but it's not about that. He wanted to do what was best for us and he wanted to be able to help us get pregnant.

For Mike and Carol, not only did they not have as many options for their epididymal sperm, they didn't have much of a choice in choosing a specialist. At that time there was only one clinic in Virginia that offered IVF. Unfortunately, they didn't get the personal touch they wanted and needed.

> CAROL: You'd call to ask questions, and you'd just get passed around. They treated you like you were a peon, that you were just somebody who came there, and they really didn't have any interest in you at all. The only person who showed any interest, oddly enough, was a nurse out there who happened to have grown up three miles from where I did. And I knew her as a girl when we were growing up in North Carolina . . . she was the only one who really showed me any genuine concern.

Mike found an increasingly competitive atmosphere that put numbers ahead of people.

MIKE: The downside of it was that we were failures and that was ruining their success rate. They had all their little flip charts with their success rates and their bar graphs and their line charts and everything. It was a business. It was a big business.

CAROL: They were cold. The push, the push, the push, you've gotta do this, you've gotta do that, and then the one thing that . . . Oh, we don't consider you a failure. If you don't have success after ten embryo transfers, then well maybe, but you've only done eight! You're not a failure! Yet!

Anne and Michael were astonished and dismayed to find that because they weren't ready to jump right to IVF, the large clinic they went to didn't make them a priority. IVF was the big-ticket item for sale there, and anyone who wasn't buying wasn't considered a prime customer.

MICHAEL: We had a very bad experience and a series of very mediocre experiences, and it seemed as though, guaranteed, no matter when you went, you were going to see a different doctor than the time before. It was a mill.

ANNE: We got zero personal attention. If you're doing IUI there, they couldn't give a crap about you. They did one IUI, [our regular doctor] did two per cycle, and I told this specialist I wanted two, and he was a real dick about it. He did it, and he'd do one, and then he'd do one thirty-six hours later. He did the first one during one of my cycles, and I don't know what he did, used a different catheter or something, and it was excruciating. It was unfortunate, because it was the first time, after [my husband and my] fight, and it was the first time he actually came in with me, and he was very squeamish. I was screaming, I was crying, it was horribly painful. I don't know what they did. They did something wrong, and [the doctor] looks up from between my legs and says, "So maybe you won't do two next time." We never went back. That was the last cycle and I was like, "Fuck you, I hate you!" That was the most obnoxious, insensitive comment you could possibly . . . it was just horrifying to me.

Finding the right physician for you is as important as the decision to do IVF at all. I really believe that our experience was as easy as the procedure allowed because we felt that we were being taken care of in the best possible sense. Everyone has different criteria for care. Some like the comfort of a large, proven facility, while others want to be coddled.

Given that you may be spending thousands and thousands of dollars on however many cycles of IVF you try, you might as well shop around. You'd do the same for a car, right? And IVF may be driving your life for quite a while. Some couples will consult with several different doctors before they find the right fit. It's definitely worth the time when you're looking at the emotional and financial commitment that is IVF.

CHAPTER 4

PAYING THE PRICE

On May 14, 2001, New Jersey Senator Robert Torricelli introduced a bill in Congress called the Fair Access to Infertility Treatment and Hope Act of 2001. The bill stated:

(a) IN GENERAL—A group health plan, and a health insurance issuer providing health insurance coverage in connection with a group health plan, shall ensure that coverage is provided for infertility benefits.

(b) INFERTILITY BENEFITS—In subsection (a), the term "infertility benefits" at a minimum includes—
   (1) diagnostic testing and treatment of infertility
   (2) drug therapy, artificial insemination, and low tubal ovum transfers
   (3) in vitro fertilization, embryo donation, assisted hatching, embryo transfer, (etc.)
   (4) any other medically indicated nonexperimental services or procedures that are used to treat infertility or induce pregnancy.

The bill would have been the answer to many Americans' prayers. With the cost of IVF ranging anywhere from $4,000 to $10,000, never mind advanced procedures like ICSI and then freezing eggs, many couples are left on the outside of a cure, looking in at what might have been. Unfortunately, this bill never made it out of the Senate. Mr. Torricelli's office said it was attached to another bill that didn't survive, and the pressure was simply not high enough to continue.

By the year 2002, fifteen states (including New Jersey) had laws on their books requiring health plans to pay for at least some infertility procedures. Some insurers allow only three tries, some fewer. My health plan paid zero. In the end, without the federal law, our bill, with ICSI and frozen embryos, amounted to $12,000 cash. Was it worth it? Yes. Absolutely. Every penny of it. Was it fair? I don't think so. I think it was highway robbery.

The reasoning behind the lack of coverage for IVF is that it is considered an "elective" procedure. In other words, you don't *have* to do it. It falls under the same category as a face-lift. I still don't understand how the government can consider infertility as not an illness. It is certainly not life threatening, except of course to potential life. But infertility is arguably a medical malfunction, and, as such, should be covered like any other malady. Some would argue that it doesn't cause any pain, so it doesn't need to be fixed; I beg to differ.

My husband and I were lucky. We both had good jobs at the time, so we didn't have to bear a major financial burden. We weighed what we had against what we wanted and decided that we were willing to try three times. The good news was that we didn't have to find out what we'd do if three tries weren't enough. Carol and Mike did.

MIKE: I dropped $75,000.

CAROL: We did two ICSIs and a second transfer from frozen embryos. We said, "There's no more money!"

MIKE: So he [the doctor] said, "We have a good relationship with the bank next door, we'll help you refinance your house."

CAROL: And then he proceeds to say, "Well, if you don't like this option, if you don't want to take some more of your own, why don't we try with donor eggs?" That's $30,000! We got up and walked out.

MIKE: That's it.

CAROL: We had $25,000 left.

MIKE: And I wasn't going to spend the last $25,000. I said we have to have $25,000 left as a reserve in case we decide to adopt kids. We've got to have a reserve.

Mike and Carol actually considered moving to France, where the government covers fertility procedures. It was more than a passing thought.

As for the teacher and the fireman, you probably know where I'm headed. Chris and Kate had no insurance coverage, and in the end, finances forced them to make their final decision. For them, right from the start, money was a cruel master.

CHRIS: The only time I felt anything against the doctor we were with, at times when [we] were just getting so discouraged, just for a brief moment it would pop into my head, you know every time they have to redo one of those tests, ka-ching, it's money out of my pocket. I don't think I would have felt this way if it was all insured, but it wasn't. We were really feeling the hit every time she had to have another test done or have another procedure.

Insemination was covered. IVF was not at all. Samples weren't covered. Once it was established what was wrong, nothing else was covered.

Chris and Kate had already spent a thousand dollars out of pocket before they even began IVF, and when they went to that first informational seminar at the fertility specialist's office, they knew they were going to be in for it.

KATE: It was broken down into how much it would cost at the seminar. Twelve to fifteen thousand.

CHRIS: They had different option packages, like you could do a one-shot deal. If you want to do it once it's nine thousand, but for twelve thousand five hundred you get two attempts or three attempts, you know, it was kind of piggybacked like that.

I felt like it was a gamble. We really had to weigh what can we afford and what are our odds. I was actually thinking, okay, if we bypass the fallopian tube, Kate is a healthy woman, you know, I think we've got great odds.

KATE: You're always thinking about money, you can't help but think about it. I was making $30,000. Chris was making about $29,000. We owned our own house, but we did not have the money.

CHRIS: So we did a home equity.

KATE: We actually credit-carded the first time. They told me I could do this mini-thing that wasn't full-blown IVF.

You use less drugs and you don't have to be on them as long, so it wasn't $9,000, it was $6,000. We put that on a credit card. What happened was I didn't have enough follicles, or they weren't stimulated enough and so we didn't get to the retrieval part.

After that, the money talk was harder. They had taken a gamble with that first try and lost—$6,000 without ever even getting to an embryo, without even doing IVF. They were already in debt but still determined.

KATE: Money was an issue, so we decided to take a little break, take some time off from the whole...
CHRIS: We needed to plan for it a little bit. Financially we had to come up with a game plan, because I had refused to think too far ahead on it, with the optimistic outlook you know, "We're going to get pregnant this time, and then this time."
KATE: And the clinic said well if you pay this much you get three cycles, or this much you get one cycle, so then we kept thinking, well where are we going to get the money, number one, and number two, did we want to pay for three cycles? If you get pregnant the first time, they'll give you 80 percent back or if you get pregnant the second time you get 50 percent back . . . you know it's just weird, it's so weird that they have this . . .
Our doctor, he was very aware of our finances; we were pretty up front with him from the get go, and he said, "Chris and Kate, I'm looking for programs to get you into." He tried to get us grant money, and ultimately what we

ended up doing was we refinanced the house, and we came up with the money on our own.

I remember several late-night discussions. At that time I was ready to call it quits, and Kate said, "You know, I don't know about this" and then she came back and said, "Let's go for it, let's do it again." And I was on board, but . . .

KATE: But then again it was like, should we pay for three cycles or one? We want to be optimistic, so it should just be one, it's going to happen, and if it doesn't happen, then we're done.

CHRIS: And that would kill our pocketbooks, that would have been a real financial trick to go with the big package.

KATE: It was like $26,000 or something like that, which was just insane.

CHRIS: Everybody in our families had their own problems.

KATE: Especially after September 11.

CHRIS: With job losses and investment losses in the market. And you know I felt like this is our problem and . . .

KATE: And we'll come up with it on our own.

CHRIS: We're adults. We can handle our own financial issues. And we did all right by the house that we purchased when we got married. We were able to pull a lot of equity out of it. Later on we were able to sell it and do well, so financially at the time, it worked out.

KATE: So we went ahead and paid for one cycle for the end of February that year.

Most of the other couples I spoke with either had some or complete insurance coverage or were independently wealthy enough to pay on their own. Because of the financial demands of IVF, it thrives in the world of the upper-middle class. For others in less fortunate positions, it is just not an option, or it's a once-in-a-lifetime chance— one chance for a life.

There are, however, stories of those who make huge sacrifices. One couple I spoke with was terrified after two tries that the third wouldn't work. Their insurance paid for only three tries, and they couldn't afford it on their own. Imagine the added stress to IVF of limited attempts!

The stories are as sad as they are egregious. I've heard of people's marriages splitting up over the financial strain of IVF. I read about one couple in England who had to sell everything they owned to pay off the debt incurred through IVF and then had to move in with their parents just to survive.

I knew a young woman in Dallas who took out a second mortgage on her house and gathered every last dime she had for one chance at IVF. When it didn't work, she told me she didn't know what made her angrier, the fact that God wasn't giving her a child or that the U.S. health care system wasn't giving her a chance.

Another couple actually considered moving to a state that required coverage. It was just that important to them that they were willing to pick up, move homes, change jobs, completely uproot their lives just for the opportunity to *try* to have a child.

There is no easy fix for the financial problems surrounding IVF. Many people look to their families for help, take out loans, or opt for the money-back-guarantee offers. But there is no guarantee with IVF and no real alternative once cheaper methods are exhausted.

THE PROCESS

CHAPTER 5

THE DRUGS

The first time I visited Alexandra at her home in Georgetown, she showed me her beautifully decorated nursery: the white wood glider, the changing station, the shelves stacked with sterling silver Tiffany rattles and shiny silver spoons. Then she took me around the house, expounding on the merits of the Pack 'N Play, the microwave steam sterilizer, the bottle organizer, the bouncy seat, the ExerSaucer, the breast-feeding pillow. I can't even remember everything. But I do remember the last thing she showed me: an album of artistic photographs—pictures of drugs. Drugs. Tiny bottles lined up in rows next to artfully placed syringes and alcohol swabs. They looked like they should be hung in a SoHo gallery for some "arts against drugs" benefit. How strange that in these odd pictures, those IVF drugs, weapons of mass production, looked almost beautiful. And Alexandra was very proud of them.

> ALEXANDRA: I was like, we have to take this photograph, because if this turns into a baby, like . . . it was just so crazy to me that this equals baby. I kept saying child-in-a-vial because we had all these vials of drugs.

PETER: We were wondering if our child was going to be born with Pyrex written on its forehead.

The drug protocols for IVF are often different, depending on which doctor you choose, but in its most basic form, IVF is about a six-week process during which time a woman's ovulatory cycle is literally taken over by her doctor through the use of various drugs. Because the science is so exact, these drugs have to be specifically measured and administered with a needle. In other words, you can't just pop an easy pill and be done with it.

First there is stimulation of the ovaries with drugs to produce multiple eggs, ovarian monitoring throughout that one cycle, more drugs to prevent ovulation, and then more drugs to prepare the eggs for retrieval. Then there is egg retrieval, fertilization, and embryo transfer. In other words, the woman is given lots of drugs to make lots of eggs and then more drugs to make sure the eggs stay where they are and then make sure they're ready to be taken out. The eggs are then removed, hooked up with sperm either naturally or through injection, and then put back in. Then the woman has to take more hormones for about two weeks to help the embryo attach to the uterine wall, which it would do naturally in regular conception. Hopefully, all of that makes a baby, or two or three or four.

Some women find the prospect of taking all these drugs terrifying. I have one friend who, after two years, still won't try IVF because she's afraid of giving herself the shots. I won't lie. It hurts, but it doesn't hurt as much as getting a negative result on a pregnancy test.

Our little home pharmacy came in three large, white paper bags. There were boxes of Lupron and Follistim, which are the drugs that stimulate the ovaries. The Follistim came in a powder that had to be mixed with sterile water, so there were tiny vials of water too. There was one megadose of hCG (Human Chorionic Gonadotropin), which is given to produce final egg maturation right before the retrieval. In no time at all, I became quite the little chemist. There were syringes, alcohol swabs, and Band-Aids. And then there was the pill. Try that on for irony. Apparently, many protocols use the birth control pill at the beginning of IVF to manipulate the female cycle exactly. I couldn't decide whether to laugh or cry, so I just swallowed hard.

Most specialists offer classes for IVFers on how to use the drugs. Some people have told me that they find this method too impersonal; because of the large group, they are often too shy or intimidated to ask as many questions as they need. We had a private session with our doctor's IVF nursing team, which I found very reassuring. They taught us, slowly and methodically, how to mix, measure, and inject. Much to my surprise, I was calm. Maybe it was just that I was finally being proactive, after all the waiting and wondering. I felt relatively certain that I could do this without a problem; I'm not particularly afraid of needles, and my brother, who has diabetes, has been giving himself shots every day since he was twenty. I would be fine with this.

The nurse suggested my husband, Scott, could give me the shots if that would be easier. In the first decades of IVF, you had to have someone else give the shots because they were done in the buttocks—intramuscularly, if there's such a word. Now most protocols have improved, and you can just give yourself the shots in the fat of your thighs or stomach. Still, like most of the women I spoke with, Kathy wanted her husband, Tim, involved.

KATHY: He was the bartender.

TIM: I was the bartender. I mixed up the drugs for her and I loaded the needles.

KATHY: All I had to do was stick myself and put it in, which was fine. It was kind of like, you have to do it at a certain time every night, so I did it a couple of times by myself, but it was better, as a routine, to have him do the mixing and then me just do the injecting.

TIM: It was kind of like an appetizer before dinner. Do the shot and have dinner.

KATHY: It was like a whole routine at night. It would have been so bad if he had been at his new job, and I would have been by myself doing everything.

Anne and Michael felt the same way. It was her way of keeping him a part of the process. I got the feeling it was also so she wouldn't have to throw a book at him again. This was a daily reminder to stay with it.

MICHAEL: I think I did all the shots.

ANNE: I called him Dr. Kildare at the end. I didn't even know how to do it. I didn't know how to mix it. He did all of it.

MICHAEL: It was a good wake-up call.

ANNE: I wanted him to be a part of it.

MICHAEL: She started out giving herself the shot, and that was one of the more dramatic changes. She went from queasiness around the needle to just being ready to be the pincushion. Then I started. It forced involvement, but that was a good thing.

ANNE: I used to hate having blood taken. Doesn't bother me at all now. I hated needles. They don't bother me at all now. Hated surgery. Walk in the park. I used to say, "I spent more time in stirrups than the U.S. Equestrian Team." I used to hate going to the gynecologist, it was just a hideous experience, now I'm fine. It's amazing what you can get used to.

Carol and Mike didn't have a choice.

MIKE: I was giving the shots.

CAROL: They wanted them in the back hip, so I couldn't do it.

MIKE: On Wednesday and Thursday nights when she had choir rehearsal, I'd go over and we'd find some excuse to go into her office, she'd drop her pants and I'd give her a shot. The kids played with the dog while I was giving her a shot. You hated it.

CAROL: Well, yeah, the first cycle was so absolutely awful because of the Lupron.

MIKE: It was something we had to do, but she really objected to the drugs. She really objected to what was happening to her body, and I did too. I don't like drugs. I don't take drugs unless I am absolutely dying. I'll take aspirin if I feel bad, but that's about it.

For some couples I spoke with, just fitting the drugs into a demanding career schedule was a feat in itself. Remember, IVF is more often than not a remedy for older women who are not as fertile anymore—older women with high-powered careers.

One woman I interviewed was a major publishing executive in New York who had to juggle business travel with shot schedules. Someone would schedule a meeting in another city, and she immediately had to consult her ovulation calendar. She talked of taking drugs on airplanes, actually going into airplane bathrooms and feeling like some kind of addict as she set up her little bottles and syringes, praying that the flimsy "occupied" lock wouldn't fail her. One time she found herself in the bathroom at Lincoln Center with all her little syringes sitting out on the holders where you throw away your sanitary pads. She had to use all kinds of public bathrooms to give herself shots. Just imagine the picture.

I chose to be my own junky. Not that I don't adore and admire my husband, but he's not exactly Mr. Handy. I figure any guy who can't hammer a nail straight into a wall shouldn't be going near me with a needle.

This is not to say that I didn't want him there. The first time I gave myself the shot I wanted him standing right next to me, not touching, but watching. I have to admit that part was pure evil. I wanted him there for support, but for some reason I also wanted him to feel some of the pain. I don't know why I would feel this way. I'm not a mean person, and I'm not big on inflicting guilt. I just didn't want him downstairs, enjoying a ball game on TV, while I was shooting up. We had to be in this together, all of it.

The first morning went fine, but the second morning I saw a little blood and pulled the needle out too quickly. A tiny drop of the drug dripped out, and I worried that I hadn't gotten the right dose. In a total panic, I called my brother at six in the morning. He was my needle expert. He reassured me that it's okay for the shots to bleed every now and then and I shouldn't panic, but I don't know that this feeling of panic ever went away.

As the days went on, the shots grew more and more routine, but I still made Scott watch me do it. I often felt angry if he didn't show up in the bedroom at the appointed time (*exactly* the same time every night even though the nurse said it could just be around the same time). When I think back on it now, I realize that it was probably harder for him to watch me than it was for me to get pricked. I deeply regret that I made him stand there like that, although to this day, I've never actually apologized. I've never even brought it up until now.

As for the drugs, I think I was lucky that I had no real reaction that I could notice outright. It was only toward the end of the cycle, after I was on the Follistim, that my ovaries really started to let me know they were filling up.

I can't say that I worried about what the drugs were doing to me physically; I just wanted them to do what they were supposed to do and make babies. But drugs treat each person differently, and Anne, who had read and studied everything having to do with fertility drugs and IVF, was surprised to find they had the worst effects on her *after* she was done with them.

ANNE: I never suffered from crushing depression before. Now I do. I have PMDD (premenstrual dysphoric disorder), so I get this horrible depression with my period each month. It's taken me two years to physically feel good again. I'm not the same person I was before we did this. It wasn't the IVF so much as the whole process. I don't feel that, even with all the stuff I read, that the doctors or the anecdotal evidence that I uncovered were very honest because of what those fertility drugs can do to you, like mess up your brain and your brain chemistry and your reproductive hormones in general. My migraines are much much worse now. I'm absolutely convinced that that's from all the fertility drugs.

There are studies that show increased risks of cancer associated with taking fertility drugs, and Carol and Mike considered that strongly before and after they did IVF. Carol was taking drugs when they underwent artificial inseminations with donor sperm, hoping to improve her chances by producing multiple eggs. Then, once they were given the opportunity to use Mike's epididymal sperm through IVF, they considered the drug factor again. They had to do IVF several times, and that factored into their decision as to when enough would be enough.

> MIKE: It was something we talked about because some of the reports were starting to come out, saying that there could be negative long-term effects of taking the Lupron and there could be some serious problems with uterine cancer, greater risks for uterine cancer. That was one of the things we talked about . . . were we going to take the risk with Carol's body, and we came to the unanimous decision that we weren't.
>
> CAROL: It was both of us at that point. It was just, I don't know how many drugs I took, but they do a number on your emotions too, and physically, just because I hurt so bad.

As I said, I didn't have any side effects from the drugs, and despite the warnings, I felt it was worth it. Most of the women I spoke with did not have nearly the repercussions that Anne did and agreed it was worth a shot, literally. I also didn't anticipate doing IVF more than three times, and somehow, at the time, as ridiculous as this may sound, living without a child seemed worse to me than living with cancer.

CHAPTER 6

POTENTIAL PARENTS: MARRIED TO IVF

My husband's urologist told him that when two people are trying unsuccessfully to conceive a child, no matter who has the actual physical malfunction, infertility is always the woman's problem. There are no fertility drugs designed for men. A man can have surgery to clear out blockage in his plumbing, but other than that it's really up to the woman to cure a couple's infertility, even if she is 100 percent functional. This may be why many of the women I spoke with felt that they bore the burden of IVF more so than their husbands, not just physically, but emotionally as well.

The biggest fight my husband and I ever had was over when we should start trying to get pregnant. Yet another of the great ironies in our quest for kids. I was standing in front of the Capitol on a very warm April day, waiting for some congressperson to finish selling some issue, while I tried to sell Scott on kids. I can't remember exactly how it started, but I had decided to go off the pill that month, and to my surprise, he objected.

We had been married just a year, but I was thirty-three and very aware of the clock. We both wanted kids very much and had talked about starting our family after a year of marriage, but because we had just moved to Washington and Scott was launching his business, he wanted to wait. So there I was on a cell phone, in a heightened but hushed tone, sure that my marriage was over, trying to convince Scott that getting pregnant may take some time, so we shouldn't delay. I have never been so right.

Like many men, Scott had a momentary bout of cold feet about being a father. Responsibility reflux, I guess. That afternoon, he ended up having a random conversation with a coworker, who is a father of two. They did a little male bonding, and by the time I got home that evening, the table was set with take-out sushi (my favorite), candles, and a repentant Scott. He was sorry, and he was ready.

We did start trying that April, but we wouldn't see our children for two more years. Those were two of the most difficult years of my life, but, in the end, I think our marriage came out better than ever. We were on equal footing, participating together every step of the way. Scott clearly felt terribly guilty that I had to go through so much when the fertility issue was his, but despite that, we did surprisingly well, at least during the process. This wasn't the case for so many others.

Most of the women I spoke with found IVF surprisingly isolating. No matter how much support their husbands gave, they were in the spotlight because they were on the drugs and on the table. As I've already said, many couples make the drug regimen a team effort, but even that can be a double-edged sword; the day-to-day task of giving injections helped some men feel more involved, but for the women, having their hormones manipulated medically didn't exactly help them cope with all the difficult emotions involved in doing IVF.

Infertility is hard on a marriage. Let me say that again: infertility is hard on a marriage, and although IVF is a treatment for infertility, it does not treat a marriage too kindly. The couple may feel like they are finally being proactive, but each will harbor emotions that are not always revealed. Some men feel left out and guilty. Some women feel angry at having to bear the brunt of the treatment. Both are scared, hopeful, and most of all disappointed that they don't get to conceive a child the way they had always planned.

That may have been the hardest part for me. I had all these visions of how we would get pregnant. There would be this great romantic night, with location changes depending on which season I was having the particular fantasy. It would be an evening we would remember and embellish for the rest of our lives. Years later we would tell our children that we made them in a chalet high in the Alps or in a secluded cove on a tropical island. "Mommy and Daddy wanted you so much that we picked an extra-special place to make you." Our child would hang on every word and make us tell the story over and over again. Each time, we would add something new, some little detail to make it that much more exciting.

How would it sound to say: "Mommy and Daddy hired some doctors to make you in a laboratory"? Where was the romance in that? Where was the warmth? Where was the love? We simply had to come to terms with the fact that the most loving thing we could do in our marriage would turn out to be an extramarital affair. Love in a petri dish. Not so simple.

So we made do, like so many others, and tried to make IVF as joint an effort as possible. Many men have a lot of trouble feeling emotionally connected to this very sterile method of conceiving a child. The process of injections at least gets the man doing something tangible, and most couples agree that sharing as much of the experience will help alleviate at least some of the isolation a partner could feel; the drugs can, as I said, serve as a bonding agent, helping the men to feel more involved.

One husband told me that what changed for him during the drug process was his having a sense of responsibility for the success or failure of it and not feeling like he was just waiting this out, and letting science take its course. He really felt that it was the turning point: he had a job, and if he didn't do it right, there was a potential life at stake. He actually practiced injections on an orange just to get the pressure right. This was recommended by one of the nurses. But he really felt that something was finally riding on his shoulders, while before it all seemed abstract.

Kate was petrified of injections, which is why she became a teacher instead of a nurse; cruel irony, right?

KATE: The first time I had to do it, he was at work, and you know, I quit nursing school because I didn't want to give anyone else a shot, and now I had to give one to myself. The first one, I called him on the phone and I made him hold on while I gave the injection to myself because I was terrified, I was really afraid; I was like, "I'm not going to be able to do it," and he's like, "Yes you are." So I put the phone on the counter, and I did it, like, "Phew!" And then later times, when he was at home, he kept wanting to give me the shots, and I said no. I just trusted myself better. It came down to a control thing.

CHRIS: After we had been optimistic through the first IVF, then on to the second, she started getting worn out.

KATE: I was a big baby, I was crying while I was giving myself a shot, like, "Oh it hurrrts."

CHRIS: And I did get to give her lots of the shots, when they had to go in her backside. At least I felt a little bit more a part of the process, and I think that was a big part of it. I wanted to share some of the experience, not the pain but at least mentally I was there. But I hated seeing her have to do all that. I thought it was very unfair that she was the one who carried the burden really. I felt sorry for her because she wanted it so badly that she was willing to do this to herself despite all her feelings about doing the shots. It killed me to see what she was going through, so the second she said, "I'm tired," I said, "Okay, you know what, we're done."

KATE: That wasn't until we did IVF again.

The shots may have been weakening Kate, but they were only strengthening her relationship with Chris, and that's no small accomplishment. These shots aren't just filled with fertility drugs, they're filled with a host of emotional carcinogens, like anguish and guilt and fear and blame and anger and self-pity. Keeping the side effects of those at bay is, to say the least, a challenge.

CHRIS: There were frustrations . . . the clinic sent her lab work out to the wrong place, and I got charged $600 more than I should have, things like that. I started getting really cynical about the process.

KATE: Certainly the stress of it added stress to our relationship, and sure, we weren't hunky-dory and happy as can be all the time, but it never was an issue where we were fighting.

CHRIS: It was always our problem together. We were our own little team.

In the beginning, Mike and Carol also felt like they were going to the same place, but their road was so long that it inevitably took a toll on their marriage. They had had so many procedures, then used donor sperm, then gone through Mike's operation, then back to IVF.

MIKE: It definitely did not bring us closer. It was tough. I sometimes wonder whether we've truly recovered from it.
CAROL: I was angry at the world and at them [the doctors]. It wasn't him. It wasn't his fault.
MIKE: There was one time you told me, how I could be such a dumb shit and volunteer and go into the army and get myself beat up. I remember that night.
CAROL: It's a roller-coaster and you just think, "Oh, this is going to work. We're going to be lucky this time. It's going to work." And then it didn't.

For Alexandra and Peter, this polarizing process brought them closer together.

PETER: I didn't feel left out, but I also felt that I didn't want to be any more a part of it than what I was. I may have been a little negligent in that respect, but I didn't get the sense. It was just hard for me to keep track of what was going on.
    It wasn't powerlessness because, no, I don't think that makes much sense because I wouldn't feel like I would have power otherwise, what can you do otherwise? You can do your part to get your wife pregnant.
ALEXANDRA: Peter was very much on board and helped, re-minding, we should probably go do your shots right now. I

couldn't get those bubbles out, so he always mixed my needles, and so he was very much like super-duper team member, in terms of schedules, like tomorrow morning we have to get up at six because I have to go to the hospital.

PETER: There were a lot of injections, but I didn't want to inject . . . because I don't like to plunge a needle in another person, much less Alexandra's thighs.

ALEXANDRA: The drugs made me moody. I cried a lot.

PETER: A lot of those things didn't affect me so much because I wasn't going to the hospital every other morning. Thank God we lived across the street from the hospital, but you know, getting things together to go there that morning and missing some of your work and the anxiety over that . . .

ALEXANDRA: And then me going and finding I wasn't responding [to the drugs], and I am running home in tears . . .

PETER: That's right, all the anticipation . . . But when you say affect your marriage, it was something we had to deal with, our relationship, but it wasn't necessarily a negative effect.

ALEXANDRA: In the end we were so much closer, a year into that, and we noticed it. I was so much more in love with him, and we were so much more, kind of a team.

When we first went to see Dr. Sacks he gave us this thick, blue folder filled with all the information we would ever need to know about the process of IVF: drug protocols, sample calendars, and definition sheets of medical terminology. Tucked in the back of the folder was one more page, an advertisement of a sort. It was for a psychologist, down the hall from Dr. Sacks, who specialized in treating patients going through IVF—a couples therapist. When I first saw the ad, I didn't think much of it. We had a marvelous, open, active relationship. We talked about everything and were constantly sharing our feelings. We definitely didn't need to see a therapist. Okay, maybe we did.

I think part of the reason I wrote it off so quickly was that I don't particularly believe in therapy, unless there is some medical, chemical imbalance that needs treatment. I've always found the idea of paying someone to listen to me pour out my feelings kind of, well, if not pathetic then maybe just embarrassing. I've also always felt that I could handle just about anything myself. I had spent a lot of time alone, traveling the country for my work and living in places where I knew just about no one. I always considered myself a very strong person overall. I'd had my share of disappointments, breakups, emotional trauma, and I'd always been able to rally, always been able to talk myself through the bad times and survive. I also always relied heavily on my friends and family as emotional outlets. Long-distance carriers nationwide love me.

IVF was different, and I should have recognized that. This was something between my husband and me, something I couldn't, or at least didn't, feel comfortable sharing with family and friends. Even though they knew what we were doing, they weren't able to say, "Here's how we handled this, that, and the other when we went through IVF."

Looking back, I wonder if we shouldn't have paid a visit or two to the woman down the hall from Dr. Sacks. Maybe I wouldn't have done some of the things I'm not so proud of, such as making Scott watch me take every shot. Maybe she could have prepared us a little better for an IVF pregnancy and for the arrival of IVF children, both of which were nothing like I expected. I know of another couple battling infertility and seeing a therapist, and it's helping them. They are saying things to her that they were unable to say to each other. I shouldn't have written it off so quickly.

Scott and I survived IVF, and I say, "survived" because that's the best word to describe it. Luckily I didn't have any emotional side effects from the drugs, so things remained about as calm as they could under the circumstances. We definitely felt closer to each other, probably because we were doing something very major and telling very few people about it. Our daily routines were completely changed. We thought and talked about nothing else. For six weeks, we shut ourselves out of social events and saw very little of our friends. Our new best friends were the nurses at our specialist's office. Our new social calendar revolved around blood tests. Our new entertainment was watching the sonogram screen. We were in this intense cocoon, going it alone, together.

CHAPTER 7

YOUR SECRET

The first news assignment I ever turned down was the biggest story I'd ever seen. It was the biggest story this country had ever seen. It was September 11, and it was during my IVF.

After a long month of drug injections and daily blood tests, our moment of truth had come. The eggs had been retrieved, fertilized, and transferred back into my body on Saturday, September 8. Dr. Sacks told me I could go back to work, but he warned me to take it very easy, I wasn't to be too active and I definitely had to keep the stress level low. He wanted the optimal environment for those embryos to do their work and attach to my uterus. I don't know that there's any data to support it, but many people think stress has a lot to do with infertility.

I had followed his orders to the letter that Monday. Congress tends to use Monday as a travel day anyway, so I came in late, took a long lunch, and went home early. Tuesday morning, as I was blow-drying my hair, I saw the "Breaking News" logo flash on the *Early Show*. Bryant Gumbel was interviewing some woman by phone about a plane crash. Minutes later, right on my little bedroom TV, I saw the second plane crash into the World Trade Center.

As a television journalist, there was little lag time in my reaction. When you see news, you go, even if you don't know where you're going. I screamed downstairs to Scott to turn on the TV, and, in a matter of seconds, I was out the door, half a head of hair still damp.

I was already down the block when I heard Scott shouting after me. He was standing barefoot on the sidewalk in front of our house screaming, "Get back here!"

"You can't go," he said.

"What? Do you see what's happening?"

"Yes, that's why you need to get back here. You can't be running around! What about the eggs? Did you forget about the eggs? You could be pregnant!"

I have to admit, for a moment, I did forget. It was the first time in months that IVF was not front and center. My mind was reeling with other possibilities. Where would I go, what would I do?

I stood for a moment in a panic. I couldn't go. I had to go. I couldn't fly to New York. I couldn't stand on my feet all day. I couldn't stay up all night. I couldn't be stressed out in any way. If I did, I could ruin everything we'd been trying so hard to get for so long. I could hurt my children. I could kill them.

"Okay, I promise I won't leave the bureau. I'll stay in DC, and I'll just help produce the coverage. I won't move, I promise."

I left Scott standing there on the sidewalk, barefoot, angry, and terrified. As I headed for a cab, trying with every reflex I had not to run, I thought, how am I going to do that? How am I going to sit still when the news is going full speed? How am I going to turn away from the story of the century? How am I going to do this without everyone at work knowing I was doing IVF?

Fortunately, I had told my bureau chief, my direct boss in Washington, about the IVF. Unfortunately, I had told no one else. The reason I told Janet was twofold: she was a friend and a mentor, and it helped me emotionally to tell her what I was doing. I also told her for very practical reasons. I was unsure of how the drugs would affect me physically. I also knew that the blood tests would make me late for work in the morning, so I felt it was important for her to know that this could affect my work for a few weeks. She couldn't have been more supportive.

I'm not sure why I didn't tell anyone else. Probably because it was none of their business and more probably because I was afraid it wouldn't work, and I didn't want the added pressure of others waiting to hear the results. We already had enough on our shoulders.

When I arrived at the bureau, it was chaos. The plane had just hit the Pentagon, correspondents were phoning in reports from the highways, and there was a buzz that something was going on with a plane in Pennsylvania. I rushed into the main newsroom, and the senior producer barked at me to jump on the FAA conference call and monitor what was happening. Perfect, I thought to myself, I'll just sit on the phone call and hide out.

Hide out. Let me just try to describe how bizarre that is. When you're a journalist, you run into things, not away from them. I have driven into forest fires, chased hurricanes up the coast, and flown thousands of miles into a war zone. I don't hide out. But I was in the critical stage of IVF, and it was a secret. No one could know, and therefore no one could understand.

About an hour into the FAA call, another buzz started that a plane was headed for the Capitol. Again, my senior producer, Jimmy, turned and barked at me. He wanted to send me to a building across the Mall from the Capitol, where we had an anchor site. From there, we had a perfect view of the dome. We could see the plane hit, we could see it hit live.

I hesitated. I paused. I looked away from his frantic eyes and said, "Can you send Sharyl?"

She was the only other correspondent not assigned.

"I'm sorry," I said. "I'll explain later, but please, just let me just stay on the call for now."

Jimmy was incredulous, but he didn't have time to think or argue about it, so he sent her, and I stayed put. Months later, when I was finally ready to tell everyone that I was pregnant, I told Jimmy first. He admitted that he thought, later, that I might be pregnant. Either that, he said, or I had lost my mind. I still didn't tell him about the IVF.

But I wasn't pregnant that day, at least, not to my knowledge. I was potentially pregnant, and when you're doing IVF, that's more precarious than actually being pregnant. It just seems like there is so much more at risk: your health, your hope, and your future child's very existence. Miscarriage is a terrible thing to happen to anybody, but to me, a miscarriage after IVF would be ten times worse. You can't just jump in the sack and try again.

So on the biggest news day our country has seen in decades, this journalist sat inside, on the phone, hiding out.

Is it best to keep IVF a secret? There are as many theories on that one as there are people doing IVF. Scott and I chose to tell our families, and I told very few friends. Scott told none of his friends until after the fact. Both of us are very close with our families and had told them all about our troubles trying to get pregnant, so it was only logical to tell them we were doing IVF. Their support throughout was invaluable. I told my one boss and a few friends . . . actually, three. Two were my closest girlfriends, and they had been suffering my whining since the start. The third was a surprise.

This woman, who prefers that I not use her name, was a friend of mine in college, but we had lost touch over the past decade and spoke probably two or three times a year. It just happened that during one of those conversations I said something about all of my friends having kids. I said I was sick of going to baby showers. She asked if I wanted to get pregnant. I said yes, and for some reason I just blurted out: "But it's harder than I thought." She was a little too silent for a moment too long, and that was when I knew she had the same problem. Suddenly a stilted conversation about our jobs, our cities, and our respective weather, gushed into a flow of hormone levels, blood tests, and ovulation predictor kits. From that day forward we spoke at least once a week. I was the only person she told, save her mother and her sister. Infertility made us fast friends again.

The same thing happened with Alexandra. She and I had gone to grade school together in New York City and then ran into each other almost twenty years later while both working as reporters in the Capitol. I immediately recognized her at a press conference; she had barely changed since the eighth grade. We exchanged pleasantries, were polite, gracious, and kept promising to get together for lunch, but never did. I'd see her at press conferences and in the House cafeteria, but that was about it. A year or so later, when Scott and I were already seeing our fertility specialist, Dr. Sacks, I heard through the grapevine that she was pregnant with twins. A friend we had in common, who knew nothing about my own fertility problems, told me in confidence that Alexandra had done IVF to get pregnant. Alexandra had only told her after the IVF was successful, and she was finally pregnant.

Scott and I were still doing IUI, but we had failed twice already and were beginning to consider IVF as a real possibility. I wanted to know everything I could about it, and I especially wanted to talk to someone who had done it. I was nervous about calling her, but more nervous about the IVF, so I sucked up my courage and called Alexandra to talk about the most personal issue in my life. We talked for more than an hour.

Alexandra has since become the guru on IVF. It's like the photographs she took of all the drugs and needles; she's just proud to show it off. Now, she tells absolutely everyone that her twins are the result of IVF, unlike when she and Peter were actually doing it.

ALEXANDRA: I felt like if I kept it secret it was less real, like less painful than if everyone knew, for some reason. It was like my new handicap, and I felt like if I just kept it in a box, you know . . .

PETER: There is a vulnerability issue, you didn't want people feeling sorry for you and asking about it every time.

ALEXANDRA: Right, I didn't want that.

PETER: And your mom breathing down your neck.

ALEXANDRA: My mom suffered to try to have me, it was just going to be so familiar to her and I just . . .

PETER: And she wanted grandchildren so bad . . .

ALEXANDRA: And she wanted grandchildren desperately, and I just couldn't take her calling me every twenty days and being like, "How are you doing?"—and it was going to be that way.

Peter told a friend at work whose wife had gone through the same thing. That was good because the guy had actually done the needles and stuff. He really knew where Peter was coming from, and it was a sense of relief, I think, for Peter. I forbade him to tell his family, and then I found out later he actually had told.

PETER: I mentioned it to Karen, my younger sister, but we never talked about it.

ALEXANDRA: I didn't want them staring at me. His brother's wife gets pregnant every time she sits on the toilet.

I just didn't want them to know anything about me. I didn't want them looking at me.

When people asked, "When are you going to have kids?" we would say, "Oh kids shouldn't have kids, we're still too young." We would just laugh it off at family reunions and stuff.

My sister and my mother were too close to me; they would've become hysterical.

I told my best friend, which ended up being very painful because she wanted to start trying to get pregnant, and now it was like a race. I wanted it first, and I have been trying harder, and if she gets pregnant before me, I am going to be crying all the time. That was a source of great anxiety.

I called Resolve [an infertility support group] and tried to get into a group, and I found it just shocking that there was no group just for women—couples only. We didn't want to do couples for the following two reasons: I will talk in front of any strange woman. I did not want to talk in front of their husbands, and Peter didn't really want to talk so much, so what we pictured happening, or at least I did, was that we were going to sit in the back, not talk, and stare at the couples and make fun of people, which is what you do when you are nervous and don't know what else to do. We would be taking notes like, well orange shirt was pretty interesting when he said this. We were going to worry about everyone else, but not get anything out of it ourselves.

Then they had a group called Women Over 40 with Diminishing Options. That was the only all-women group.

PETER: I wanted to tell people now and then, you know, to share it. It was just an occasional thing; I don't think I had a constant ongoing need for support. I kind of wanted to tell her family, but sometimes I completely understood why she couldn't. There was just no question.

ALEXANDRA: But then in vitro marked a year of fertility treatments, and if that first round of IVF didn't work, Peter thought I had to tell them.

PETER: That's right. Sometimes I really wanted to pop that safety belt, not safety belt, but kind of, you know, just let her share with people. Those were the darkest moments.

ALEXANDRA: After in vitro, I felt if this fails, I want to get an adoption lawyer, and I want to ask my dad for $50,000. I don't know if I can do in vitro again is what I said.

PETER: Because of the emotions . . .

ALEXANDRA: And the drugs. I was feeling pretty pickled at that point. I just didn't know how I would feel. Of course now I know that if it had failed, I would have waited two months, and I would have done it again, but I only know that now. The longing is really what kills you. I mean more than anything, even if it [the fertility problem] was him, me, a combination, it was the aching and the longing that was just killing me, and that was what I felt was going to be more real and more loud and reverberate more in my daily life if I shared it. If I wore it all over, because I am the most open person, then we would've never stopped talking about it.

Something about keeping it private made me live the rest of my life. It was actually good because I'd get on the phone with my mother, and I would have to talk about work, the garden, what we were doing this weekend. I would not talk about it, and I would be reminded that there were other things going on in my life. So in a way it was productive because it forced me to live in the moment of my day. I don't have a baby this weekend, I am not pregnant this weekend, what am I doing this weekend? Is this all I ever talk about and think about? It really actually was healthy in a way to compartmentalize and say, what else do I have in my life?

People say you forget the pains, as you know, it's not that much of a physically painful process. You learn to take a needle. Needles will never bother me again. The memory of lying in my bed and wanting this baby and putting the needle in and thinking okay, this looks so ugly, this seems so crazy, I'll be bouncing a baby on this bed, in this very bed, in this room, the sun will come in, I'll have babies in this house. I can remember that so clearly. A year ago today I can remember lying in my bed trying to think positive thoughts. That was the thing. If I opened up that dam, it was just going to be every time my mother called. It was

going to be "why me?" and all that stuff, which you just
think all the time.

For practical reasons, when she started doing IVF, Alexandra did
tell her direct boss. She had a very demanding job at that point, as a
Capitol Hill producer for a major television network, and she knew
she would have to make time for the blood tests and the sonograms.
Alexandra's boss, like mine, was extremely understanding and accom-
modating. Kate's boss was as well—a female principal at an elemen-
tary school was easy—but for Chris, how about telling the guys at the
firehouse that you have to spend the morning having fun with a cup?

> KATE: I had to tell her. I've got to go through IVF, and I
> have to go to the doctor in the mornings, and I have to do
> ultrasounds, and they have to do my blood, and if they tell
> me I have to take this time off . . . you know she was very,
> very understanding, and, "Whatever you need Kate, you
> get here when you get here and when you need to be gone
> that's fine. Good luck."
>
> She knew and probably about three of my friends. I
> didn't think it would be a problem. My work wasn't so
> much a source of stress, but what stressed me out was the
> fact that Chris worked twenty-four-hour shifts and then
> had forty-eight hours off, and what if that was the time that
> I needed him to meet me and he wasn't going to be able to
> because he was at work. He was only in his job a year . . .
> would he be able to get time off, would he be able to leave?
> Trying to coordinate his schedule with my body's schedule
> stressed me out.

CHRIS: That's when I finally had to tell. My chief was okay. You know, the department I was with at that time was a large department, and you could never really tell where you're going to be from shift to shift when you're new. Our battalion chief more or less said, "Well, you know, when the time comes we'll do what we can do to make it work for you."

I was fortunate I guess. My own station was a battalion headquarters, so the fire chief for our battalion was in my station and I had a good relationship with him. We had a very good family atmosphere at our station, an open-door policy. People were supportive, and at this particular time we were far enough into it that, pretty much, I was beyond it all.

Talking to friends, though, was different. There was no sense of shame for Kate or Chris, just an overwhelming fatigue. I found this to be a common thread with pretty much everyone I interviewed as with myself. You just get tired of talking about it.

KATE: It wasn't a sense of shame. I felt that it was a very personal thing, and the whole year that I was trying to get pregnant, four people that I worked with got pregnant and had those babies that next summer, so I was surrounded by people getting pregnant, being pregnant, having the babies, so it was really hard for me. They kept asking me, and I just got tired of having to tell them no, so I just said, "We're going to take a little break." I didn't want to have to deal with it.
CHRIS: It got to a point where you just didn't want to talk about it because it's something that for Kate and me it was so much a part of our lives and of all the thoughts . . . on our

minds, and you didn't want to have to tell the story to somebody. I also think in a way I was a little embarrassed, probably because of the process I had to go through to make this happen, you know go into a little room by yourself, that's the bad aspect with a touch of embarrassment, especially in a firehouse. Macho guys who would say that, "Oh, Chris has a problem . . . mm hmm." I wasn't even about to go there with anybody I worked with. Maybe it was an imaginary fear, but it was one of the things that I was feeling at the time.

I don't think anybody really cared, you know, not like Kate's friends, my friends would be like, if I brought up the topic, you know, that's an uncomfortable conversation for my friends and coworkers. I think a response to that would be, oh, okay. I think the guys looked at it as, if you said something about infertility it always reverted back to going into the little room and doing your business in a cup. It was a topic more to be made fun of. The guys, they're not sensitive to the feelings and emotions that are attached to this sort of process.

No one actually did that to me, but I didn't really tell anyone about it either. I had a fear of them doing that, and it was something I was emotionally connected to and I could see if somebody did do that it would have bothered me, so I figured, I'm not going to even go there.

KATE: It was harder for me with my friends because we all started trying to get pregnant at the same time and it was harder for me each time to find out that they were pregnant, and I still wasn't. They'd either say things to me that they thought would make me feel better or give me advice, and that was harder than being around the children and working with them every day.

CHRIS: They just said, "You need to relax."

KATE: Yeah, I just loved that one, especially when I know there's something medically wrong, and you still get this, "Well you know maybe if you just drink some wine," or "Are you laying in bed for thirty minutes after? Are you propping your legs up?" And I'm like, you don't understand, I tried that stuff for a year, now there really is something medically wrong and now we're trying other things. It's like they said what they thought I needed to hear, and I didn't need to hear any of that.

CHRIS: One of the things I remember about that time in regards to Kate was the children in her classroom, the mothers were younger than she was, and I know that was one of the things that was just a reminder to her that she was getting older. And the kids in their innocence would ask, "Why aren't you a mommy?"

KATE: And when I got a little heavy, "Are you pregnant?"

Tim and Kathy's experience with infertility was relatively short-lived, and they were always very open about it with their friends and families. But at work, in the middle of a busy Boston television station, it was another story.

KATHY: Most of the time when you do your ultrasounds and do your blood tests in the morning, I would do it before work and go in to work, but when I was scheduled for an eight o'clock shift, you just couldn't do it all.

I was being honest. "Hi, we're trying to have a baby, it's not like I don't want to get out of bed." But a new news director started at the same time that I started my treatment, and that was a problem, because once a couple of conflicts came about, you know how the procedures go, and you have to be there for the better part of a morning sometimes and then go to work, and she didn't want any part of that. She didn't want me going in late; she wanted me to take a sick day. It became a problem because I had a new boss. . . . She's one of those types who doesn't have a kid, doesn't have a boyfriend, doesn't have a life. News hag.

In the end I had to hire a lawyer. I hired a lawyer and told him to write a letter that they were violating the pregnancy act, the disability act, et cetera.

TIM: She put that in writing, and that was it. I was on the phone with the lawyer saying, "I want her boss to back down. This is bullshit!" If you look at all the appointments, dozens of appointments, and she's late for work two or three times because of medical appointments. You can't be touched for that.

KATHY: She didn't understand it, and you know what? We wouldn't have conversations about it. She's like, this is getting to be a real problem. I said yeah it is. Sometimes I'd switch with reporters who had gone through the same thing and knew—"Kath, your thing is tomorrow, yeah, no problem I'll do it." And even that wasn't good enough for her.

TIM: What was so frustrating for me is, her boss was not a man. I would have expected that from a man; never in a million years would I see this coming from a woman.

KATHY: Once we hired the lawyer, and he wrote that letter, they didn't screw around with me.

Unfortunately, this story is not all that uncommon. Carol had a similar experience at her job, yes even at a church choir, and that spilled over into her decision not to tell anyone, not even friends about what she and Mike were doing. It just plain poisoned the water. She wanted to be open and honest, but after the first negative reactions at work, she didn't want to risk any more in her personal life.

CAROL: My boss at the time was a real jerk. I had to tell him because of the procedures and having to take time off from work.

MIKE: A big discussion we had way back when was when we were using donor sperm of how open we were going to be about that, and pretty much decided that we weren't going to be open about it at all. We just have always been sort of a contained unit. We have a few good friends, but there was really no one that we were that close to of our friends that we felt any need to tell.

CAROL: You don't know if it's going to work, and you just don't need everybody asking you, and prying into your affairs all the time.

MIKE: It was such a roller-coaster for us; we didn't feel that we wanted to put our friends through that too.

CAROL: And then every time it didn't work . . .

MIKE: Then everyone would say, "Oh, that's so bad."

CAROL: Then you spend the next two months telling them that it didn't work and reliving it again every time you talk to somebody. One of the couples that we did actually talk to was one of my college roommates, only to discover that they were at the same clinic at the same time we were; they used donor sperm and they conceived.

I don't regret not telling the world. I don't think that would have been right because in the job that I have, it's almost a five-hundred-member church. I work with at least ninety people, and if you tell somebody, then they're going to tell somebody else, and then the whole church is going to know, and then everybody I walk up to and say anything to is going to know. That's private for me. I don't need that many people knowing what's going on in my life, even if they're well meaning.

And there's no one that can make you feel any better about it. It's just part of what happens. Somebody can't tell you, "I know, I know." They can commiserate, but they can't make you feel better about what's going on.

Anne would disagree, vehemently. Her aspirations to get into DC politics resulted in a job as a defense analyst with a large government contractor. She worked in a very close-knit group and got such support from her coworkers that she kept it from no one.

MICHAEL: She was telling people in supermarkets.
ANNE: My office knew what was going on. I was very close with all the people I worked with and people talked about personal stuff all the time. They were, "Take all the time you need, do what you want to do." They were amazing. I have a very unique situation. I know that that's an unusual experience.

My experience was the more people I told, the more support I got. Everybody was very sympathetic and very concerned and very supportive, very positive. I had a lot of people saying prayers for me, and you know, I'll take them. I'm not big on secrecy, and I didn't think this was anything to be ashamed of.

MICHAEL: The question is whether society is changing. At one point there was almost a stigma if it's not natural. I don't know if society is changing or we've gotten so used to the reality of IVF and the naturalness of IVF. It's not like I whisper it under my breath. I don't volunteer it to people walking by like my wife does. We've never felt like it's anything we should be ashamed of.

I did. For some indescribable reason, I still, to this day, get queasy about telling people how we got pregnant—*and I'm writing a book about it!* I even surprised myself one day at the gym. I was pregnant and showing. A trainer, whom I have known for a while, was congratulating me and asking if I knew what we were going to have. I told him that actually we had just found out it was twins. Another trainer, a woman, who overheard our conversation piped in, "Oh, did you do fertility stuff?"

Without skipping a beat, I said no. "Just luck I guess." Why did I do that? I asked myself that question all day and still do to this day. I was already researching this book at the time, talking to dozens of people about fertility, calling couples I had never met, but for some reason I didn't want this woman at the gym to know. For some reason, when it came to me, I was fiercely protective and even offended that this woman would ask me such a personal question.

The question of shame is a tricky one. I admit it: as a woman, I felt a sense of shame because I wasn't able to get pregnant immediately. Even after we learned that it was Scott's issue, I think I felt ashamed for us as a couple. I can't explain for sure why. Perhaps it was a feeling closer to embarrassment than shame. It's just a sense of being abnormal. Here is something that everyone else seems to be able to do so easily, something that is a common right of passage after marriage, and we simply couldn't do it on our own. Two well-educated, healthy, hard-working people could not produce a baby. There must be something wrong with us. There must be some reason behind it all, not medical, but something we did wrong in the past for which we were being punished or some flaw in one of our characters that made parenthood out of the question. Something or someone had judged us and judged us unfit.

Looking back, I am glad we told only the few people we did. Even though our families only wanted the best for us, knowing how much they wanted to see us have kids added to our stress. And there is really nothing anyone can say. There is no great advice, especially from someone who has never gone through it. Even people who have gone through it are tough to talk to at the time. Either they had it really easy, and you feel competitive stress, or they had it really hard, and you fear you'll end up like them.

And then there are decisions, decisions that nobody but you and your spouse should make—decisions that are so personal to your relationship that no doctor, family member, or IVF survivor can make for you. For a while, IVF is a pretty straightforward protocol. You follow the rules, take the drugs, and time the procedures—until one fateful day.

CHAPTER 8

MOVING DAY:
RETRIEVAL AND TRANSFER

Ask any man to list his ten greatest fears, and odds are he'll put "inability to perform sexually" somewhere near the top. Take the actual sexual performance question out of the equation, and you would think it would be easy, that is, to do it on your own (after all, most men have been masturbating since they were thirteen). Not necessarily the case with IVF. One man I interviewed had to face that very fear on the worst possible day.

He and his wife were going through IVF for the first time, and it was egg retrieval day. His wife had produced several viable eggs, and the retrieval had taken place very early in the morning. All he had to do was ejaculate into a cup, and the doctors would take it from there.

He couldn't do it. He tried from ten in the morning until ten at night. First in the doctor's office, they gave him magazines. Then he went home and tried it there. Then he went back to the office for one more shot. Finally, he and his wife just went home. They lay down on their bedroom floor and cried. The chance was gone, and they would have to wait and try again the next month. All the drugs, all the waiting, timing, and preparing that the woman went through were all for naught. The man was just so stressed out by the whole process that something between his brain and his—well, it just didn't connect. Apparently this is not all that uncommon.

The couple did finally end up having twins through another IVF cycle, and they laugh about it now, but imagine the stress on that horrible day! Your wife has just gone through a month of drug injections, she's just been on the table having her eggs removed, and it's all up to you to bring home the bacon. Seems easy enough, and then it suddenly seems impossible.

Our retrieval day went pretty smoothly, except that the drug cocktail they used to sedate me made me horribly sick to my stomach. My doctor gave me the option of being awake for the procedure, during which he inserts a needle through the vagina, into the uterus, and then through the uterine wall and up to the ovaries. He then sucks out the fluid that holds the eggs. I chose not to be awake. I mean . . . *why?*

So my doctor gave me a combination of Valium, Demerol, and morphine; it totally knocked me out. I remember chatting with the anesthesiologist, and then I remember waking up in recovery, feeling no pain. Unfortunately, a few minutes later I became terribly nauseated and proceeded to dry-heave for the rest of the day.

Still, the operation was a success. Scott did his duty without a problem, and while we headed home, me heaving in the front seat of the car, a technician named Sam sat at a table in a laboratory and made our children. We have never met Sam. I doubt we ever will.

Four days later we went back to the hospital and waited for Dr. Sacks. He came in with a clipboard and a whole set of numbers. Of the eighteen eggs he retrieved, twelve had fertilized. One had collapsed on itself, but the other eleven were viable. Some, however, were better than others.

Doctor Sacks explained to us a complicated rating system for the embryos, much of which is based on how many times the cells divide. The more divisions, the better.

We had several good embryos, which was very good news of course, but it put us in a position to make a very big decision. How many should we put back in?

We had discussed this beforehand and decided definitely two. We had actually asked Dr. Sacks if he would be willing to transfer only one, but he said two was his absolute minimum because he felt that the cost was too high—not the cost of the procedure, but the cost to my body with all the drugs. So we agreed we would do two, figuring that this was our first try, and if it didn't work, we would just do it again.

We told Dr. Sacks before we started IVF that we would only put two back, so we were surprised when he had a different opinion on transfer day. He suggested three. I think I stopped breathing. I definitely remember the room started to move. I had been so worried that we wouldn't get good embryos that I had trouble focusing on anything he was explaining. At one point I just said, "Do we have good ones? Can we do this?"

He was busy talking about the ratings and explaining why he thought we should try three. He said it would improve our chances for success, and if it happened that they all took, and we were averse to triplets, we could "selectively reduce." He knew a great surgeon in Pennsylvania who specialized in that.

How could we do that though? We had been trying to have children for two years. How could we abort a potentially healthy child?

Don't get me wrong, I'm as liberal as they come and 100 percent pro-choice, but this just didn't make sense. Not for us. I didn't want to even consider the option, so we made sure it would never be an option. We stood firm on two.

The transfer was totally easy and uneventful, save for the Chinese delegation. In the midst of all this grave decision making, Dr. Sacks had asked, "Oh, by the way, there's a delegation of Chinese fertility specialists who have never seen an embryo transfer. Mind if they watch?" Whatever. I'll always play to a crowd.

It was even on TV, an ultrasound monitor anyway. I tried to experience this pivotal moment, feel truly and deeply the moment when my children were deposited in my warm body for safe keeping, but frankly I couldn't tell what the hell I was looking at. Scott says he could see the catheter and watched the two embryos come out, like two little pebbles darting in. He found it surreal, hard to fathom that those little specks were the makings of life. I just saw fuzzy shadows on the screen.

I suppose it depends on your personal view of conception. It's obviously one of the greatest debates between churches and governments, but I never really knew my own opinion until I was lying on that table. There were the embryos, fully fertilized and full of the potential to be my offspring. But they had a very, very long way to go. They could either attach to the wall of my uterus and start growing, or they could just come right back out. There wasn't much I could do to keep them in, although I'll admit that for days afterward I tried not to walk too fast, step too hard, or sit too bumpily. I actually caught myself tensing up and crossing my legs more than once. Ridiculous, I know, but I swear it was almost like a reflex.

Even though I was suddenly highly protective of what was supposedly inside me, I definitely didn't consider myself pregnant, especially when I saw those fuzzy images on the screen. I didn't feel as if I were carrying life. My most basic image of getting pregnant was that my body would produce something, and eventually it would come out. There would, of course, be the introduction of a foreign body, the sperm, but, in my mind, that was really just something to help the process along. The child would be made of me. If you want to get technical, during IVF, you are nowhere near your children when they are "conceived," so, for me at least, getting them back was something like getting a pacemaker or a breast implant (not that I have either, I swear!), but something foreign inside me, something not really made of me. I think I lost contact with that natural feeling of life when the eggs were first taken away. I think that's why I never felt particularly pregnant.

After the transfer, they wheeled me back to a room on a gurney and told me to stay lying flat for two hours. Dr. Sacks admitted there was absolutely no scientific proof that lying down would help anything, but apparently it makes the hospital feel better. He called it voodoo. I mean, you can get up right after sex and still get pregnant, right?

I wasn't taking any chances. I stayed flat for two hours, holding in an enormous pee; they tell you to drink a lot of water before the procedure because a full bladder makes the uterus easier to see. Dr. Sacks did say I could go to the bathroom afterward, but I decided to wait the ridiculous two hours, fearing, of course, that I would somehow pee out the embryos.

Then we drove home very slowly, avoiding as many potholes as possible, and I got into bed to watch movies. I tried not to think about the enormity of what had just happened, and believe it or not that wasn't so hard. The whole thing was just so cold. It was science: shots, blood tests, a catheter, and blotches on a screen. To me, none of that added up to squealing pink babies. I knew I was potentially pregnant, but I didn't feel potentially anything. I had two growing embryos inside me, two future children; I should have felt exhilarated, but all I felt was tired.

Chris and Kate had been tense as well on their second try at IVF. It was the first time they actually had any eggs to use. Money was tight, and they were gambling on this one try.

KATE: I did all my shots. They told me I had eleven follicles or something like that, and we went in and they took the eggs out of me. They hoped that we could go five days and get the blastocysts, but when they called us three days later, they said, they're looking good, we're going to let them go . . . but all they got were seven eggs. Six of them looked good. Of the six, only three fertilized. Of the three, only two were usable. That was disappointing.

CHRIS: They gave us the option at the very beginning, before we knew how many embryos we had, of putting in three.

KATE: But then what if all three took? I thought, "Oh my God, no, twins were fine." I never wanted to put three in, even though I knew that would increase my chances, because I knew I wasn't prepared for that. I could handle it if we had twins, but if that third egg wasn't that great anyway.

CHRIS: I was excited about the idea of twins. I always thought I'd have two children.

KATE: And at this point you're like if we could have two at the same time, we're done. We knew it would be difficult, but it's not like we wanted to do it again. If two were meant to be then two would be okay.

Of the couples I spoke with, I was surprised to find that some were willing to transfer three and four embryos without thinking twice. Perhaps they were more desperate than we were or believed a little less in the science. None, however, said they were willing to do selective reduction. Anne and Michael really rolled the dice and put in four.

MICHAEL: We were somewhere between gutsy and naive. We spent so much time after the hCG shot [the shot that they give right before retrieval to mature the eggs], thirty-six hours in Norfolk, not a hell of a lot you can do in Norfolk in the winter, and we talked and talked about the pros and cons and listed them out back and forth.

ANNE: Our doctor's protocol for somebody under thirty-five was to transfer a maximum of three embryos. So the back and forth was whether to transfer three or to transfer two, because we felt we could handle twins but not triplets. If I had gotten pregnant with triplets, I had huge moral qualms about a reduction to twins. I didn't want to have to make the decision, and I didn't want to have triplets.

MICHAEL: We got to the hospital, and they told us that there were four or five eggs that were graded four or five.

ANNE: Of the ten, I think seven had fertilized and of those seven, four of them were twos and threes, three of them were fours and fives. One being the best, and five being the worst. Their protocol was that they didn't transfer fours and fives, unless that was all you had. The nurse, not even the doctor, they were taking blood the morning of the transfer, and she came in and she's like, "So, you just want to transfer all four?" Just like that. I was thirty-three at the time, just under thirty-four. Essentially, the argument being, it wasn't worth freezing just one, and the one you'd freeze would be a three. There's no point in freezing a three. So then, the question was, do you transfer all four or do you dump the potentially viable one. We literally had to make a decision in two seconds. So we did. We're like, yeah, what the hell, after all of that!

MICHAEL: This great moral struggle between two and three . . . so you want four? Sure!

ANNE: We turned to her and said, "What would you do?" And she said, "I'd do the four." We didn't want to talk to the doctor, only the nurse. We never met the specialist before.

MICHAEL: We weren't allowed to use that word, quadruplets, in the house. Nothing that started with Q.

ANNE: I didn't think we would get four at all. In talking to us about whether to transfer three or four, the nurse kind of made it sound like the threes just weren't that great, and you might as well put them in because probably nothing's going to happen anyway. That was my impression.

According to the 1999 CDC report "Assisted Reproductive Technology Success Rates," of all the live births resulting from ART that year, 32 percent were twins and 5 percent were triplets (more

than 8 percent of the pregnancies started out as triplets but were either "selectively reduced" or didn't survive).

Tim and Kathy knew of that risk and weighed the data carefully.
They definitely wanted their big Irish-Catholic family, but they
didn't exactly want it all at once. They got the same surprise we did,
when their doctor, like ours, walked into the room the day of their
transfer and suggested they go for broke.

> TIM: The doctor came out and he said, "We've got three re-
> ally good embryos here. I would say put them all back." My
> eyes got real wide. I'm like, three?!
>
> KATHY: When we filled out the paperwork, I probably said
> three was the most I could ever have, but I never thought
> they'd be using three. In the big picture, three was the most
> I could ever conceive, not want.
>
> TIM: He gave us some time, and we sat there going,
> "Three, three, oh my god, three, what if three caught?"
>
> KATHY: We looked at each other like, honey? Are you
> telling me? Did we miss something here? Because he's all
> gung ho for three now, the doctor.
>
> TIM: So he said, "All right, this will help you: look at the
> question from the opposite direction. What's going to be
> worse news? You're not pregnant or you're pregnant with
> three?" We're like, easy answer, pregnant with three is
> much worse than not pregnant, because that's a real good
> possibility. We looked at it like that. We could have triplets!
>
> KATHY: That's a whole life-changing . . .
>
> TIM: So we said, "How about two? We're comfortable with
> two." He said, "I would put three back, but two's good."

KATHY: He said, "I'm a betting man." But we said, "Okay, you are, but we're not."

That would be horrible, selective reduction, that sounds terrible.

TIM: To me, I have friends with twins, and I know how challenging that's been for them, and I was scared of triplets. Very scared of three babies. Just everything. All of a sudden you're sitting in a doctor's office and you're thinking, three in college? All at the same time? Eighteen years later. Your mind races through all these issues. I think we were comfortable with two.

Multiple births are a definite risk in IVF, but not always an unwanted one. Some actually want twins, so they don't have to dance with IVF more than they have to. Alexandra was so sure that her chances were limited that she was actually hoping for just that.

ALEXANDRA: So when they said to me that morning you have two really good embryos, they said, "You know we don't really usually tell people this, but it's looking very good, you want to put one in?" I was like no, put both. I said I am thirty-four, I might never get pregnant again, I'd love to have twins, and they told us what the odds were. Meaning they knew, the odds were on that it was going to work, so they were thinking, don't you just want one? The second one was for insurance. I said, "No, I want twins."

I can't say Scott and I definitely wanted twins, but we didn't *not* want them either. I think most couples who go through a long period of infertility are more willing to accept multiples because they may not be able to do IVF more than once. Age, money, and emotions all contribute to the limited life span of IVF in each couple's world. Whatever the reason, I found that of all the people I interviewed, none were concerned at the outset about the possibility of having twins. I never believed we would have two. I believe it now, but I'll get to that later.

SUCCESS?

CHAPTER 9

YES!

I'm sitting in an outdoor café in Georgetown, sipping a small latte, my twin babies napping in their side-by-side stroller, as I write this sentence. I still can't believe I got pregnant. I don't think I ever truly believed that IVF would work, any more than I believe that my twins will ever sleep through the night. Things change. Things happen. Last night, my daughter, Madeline, made it to 6 A.M.

The days after our procedure were filled with confusion. September 11 was all around us, and it was hard to think that as we watched all the stories of death and loss, that we might have just created life.

I also wasn't feeling well. I was so bloated, sore, uncomfortable, and crampy that I was sure I was premenstrual. Every day, I expected to get my period, as I had every time before. Dr. Sacks had told me that I would actually get more bloated after the procedure than before, but for some reason I thought that once my follicles were emptied, I would feel empty. Instead, as he said, they filled up with fluid, so I felt worse.

Scott and I were told we would have to wait two weeks before a blood test could show anything. I could take a home pregnancy test, but the doctor said that given all the drugs in my system, it was unlikely to be accurate either way. I debated that one for a while. I had a test stick in my medicine cabinet. What could it hurt to give it a shot? But let's not forget my usual negative attitude: if it was positive, I'd be worried that the drugs had given a false result. If it was negative, I'd be sure the test was accurate and resent the fact that I had to wait to get an official test. In other words, it was a no-win situation, so I opted not to play, even though I swear the kit called to me from the cabinet every time I walked past the bathroom. Instead we waited. Our families waited. The few friends we had told waited. I think that test stick is still in the medicine cabinet today, although I truly doubt I will ever need it again.

The days dragged, and as each one passed, I felt less and less pregnant. Perhaps it was all the physical side effects, or just the fact that for the first time in more than a month we weren't actually *doing* anything on a daily basis. There were no more injections, no blood tests, no nothing except a nasty progesterone suppository I had to use, just in case it had worked.

I come from the school of "Don't expect anything, and you won't be disappointed," so I refused to talk about the prospect of it working. There were no "What ifs?" in our conversations. I wouldn't even let myself visit the possibility, wouldn't allow one measly fantasy of how I would decorate the nursery or what type of stroller I might buy. One day, during that time, Scott asked me if I wanted a boy or a girl. To be honest, I hadn't even thought about it. I thought about it years before, when we first started trying to get pregnant, but once we learned we were infertile, it never crossed my mind again. I couldn't even visualize pregnancy, let alone children.

I could visualize failure, however, quite easily. Scott and I were scheduled to drive to Massachusetts for his sister's wedding the day after our two weeks were up, and all I could think about was how was I going to deal with such a happy occasion after I found out our IVF didn't work. My parents were coming to the wedding, so everybody was represented, everybody who was waiting for the answer, just like us. So we decided it would be best if we just lied to our families and told them we would not be tested until the Monday after the wedding. It would allow us a few days to deal with the results on our own, as a couple, and it would prevent a potential cloud from hanging over the wedding.

Then the fateful Thursday finally arrived. I walked over to Dr. Sacks's office alone and went in to have my blood drawn for the ninety-ninth time. Carol, one of his nurses who had worked closely with us, asked why I looked so glum. I told her I was crampy and bloated and sure I wasn't pregnant. She didn't say anything. At first I was a little miffed that she wasn't offering any encouragement, but looking back on it now, I realize that there was nothing she could say, nothing. She took my blood, and I walked home. The results would come the following morning.

Since we were supposed to set off for the wedding that Friday, I went to get my hair done and then hurried home to meet Pascal, a salesman from European Designs, a local cabinetmaker that was going to build us a home office. My plan for the day was to do everything I could to keep my mind off the results, even though I was sure they were negative. I walked in the door just as the phone was ringing. It was Carol.

"You can't tell Dr. Sacks I'm calling you. I could lose my job for telling you this, but I wanted you to know that we do a test here in the office before we send it out to the lab, and your hCG count is so high, that it's definitely positive."

What?!

Positive how? For a moment I had no understanding of the word positive. Did that mean yes or no?

"Pregnant!" she said. "Knocked up!"

I think I made her say it about six times before I let her hang up. She said the lab would confirm it for us, but she had no doubt in her mind that the IVF worked. I just stood there, sweating, slightly nauseated, and completely unsure of what to do. Scott wasn't home. He had his cell phone with him, but I couldn't tell him on a cell phone! For years I had been planning and fantasizing about how to tell him I was pregnant. I'd make this romantic dinner at home, and in the candlelight I'd surprise him. Or we'd go out somewhere fancy, and I'd surprise him. Or I'd take him to some beautiful spot and surprise him.

But the surprises were gone in our life. We were all about schedules, timing, injections, and tests. Scott and I had been told that we would get a phone call Friday morning, and, knowing we'd both be waiting by the phone, I gave up any thoughts of springing it on him romantically. This was business. But now I suddenly had a new chance. I could actually spring it on him. What should I do? Where should we go? I wondered how long it took to rent one of those airplanes that writes stuff in the sky?

I sat down in the middle of the living room rug. I sat down, and I thanked God. I'm not religious. I don't even know if I believe in God, but it was all I could do. It was all I could think of to do. I was in total disbelief, and I guess I figured God was the only one who could understand. I also thought it was the safe thing to do. Just to make sure it would stay true. So many thoughts and feelings were reeling through my mind that I almost didn't hear the doorbell ringing.

It was Pascal from European Designs.

I snapped back into myself, took him downstairs, and sat on the couch as he measured, talked moldings, showed samples. I had no idea whatsoever what he was talking about, but I did manage to choose a wood grain. How surreal it all was. I had this marvelous news that only Carol knew. I wanted to shout it from the rooftops, but I certainly wasn't going to let Pascal be the one to hear it first.

He went on and on and on and on. Finally, just as he was leaving, Scott came in. They chatted for a bit about wiring and fixtures, and at last Pascal was out the door. I was suddenly very calm. I still had no idea how to tell my husband that he was finally going to be a father, that our infertility was cured. We actually talked about the desk for a few minutes, which believe it or not turned out fabulously.

Then I went back upstairs to the living room, and it all started in my mind all over again. What would I say? How would I say it? Should I wait? Do it over a romantic dinner that night? How could I wait?! Forget it. The romance was gone, and I wasn't going to get it back over any expensive dinner. I called for Scott. As soon as he reached the top of the stairs, I threw my arms around him and kissed him hard on the lips.

"We're pregnant!"

"What?"

"We're going to have a baby. Carol called this morning. She wasn't supposed to, but she did, and we're pregnant."

He sat down and cried. I will never forget his face. I am not enough of a writer to describe it, but I will never ever forget it.

We went to the wedding the next day, and whispered it one at a time to each of our parents. My mother cried huge tears, more parts relief than joy I think, and my very reserved father actually gave my husband a very big hug. We didn't want Scott's sister to know until the wedding was over, as we wanted it to be her day alone, but it was a magical day for everyone. Then, on the drive home, I called the few friends who knew we were doing IVF.

Everyone was overjoyed, but for some reason I was still skeptical. I still didn't feel pregnant. The strangest thing was that a few people at the wedding actually asked my mother-in-law if I was pregnant. Apparently I was so bloated from the drugs that at two weeks I was already showing. The doctor had said it would take about two weeks for all the fluid to pass out of my system. He had even suggested I buy my bridesmaid dress one size too big. He knew what he was talking about!

It had worked. One try, and it worked. You would think I would have been thrilled. I don't think I was. I was certainly excited and nervous, but the warm and fuzzy feeling of love that I imagine most couples feel when they first find out they're pregnant was missing. Our lab experiment had worked, but somehow it didn't compute in my mind. It didn't add up to Scott and me making babies. I just couldn't see it. Again, it didn't feel natural. It's like playing the daily Lotto. You don't really expect to win. You really just expect to keep on playing.

Most of the successful couples I spoke with had a hard time actually believing they were pregnant too. Most of the women, in fact, were quite sure they weren't.

ANNE: They wait ten days to test you. I actually spent thirty-six hours on bed rest after, and then we had the ten-day wait. I had a book called *Taking Charge of Your Fertility*. I interpreted the book to read that if you were pregnant you would have a triphasic pattern, and so I was obsessively taking my temperature throughout that ten-day period. I never had it. My temperature didn't drop, like it would for my period, but it was only ten days after the transfer, so I was not even at day twenty-eight. I was absolutely 100 percent positively convinced I wasn't pregnant.

MICHAEL: She's an extremist. She will believe something on an issue, and sometimes it's an absolute yes, and tomorrow it may be absolutely no, but it's still absolute. So she was not 99.9 percent convinced she wasn't pregnant. She was 100 percent convinced she wasn't pregnant. Just couldn't be.

ANNE: The ten days after the transfer was a Friday, and they tested me and I could have sworn I had an agreement with the nurses at the office that they were going to tell me if they thought I might be pregnant. They didn't say anything, so I spent the weekend literally grieving. My journal is filled with, "Okay, it didn't work this time. We'll do it again in two months because you have to take a month off."

And I was at peace with it not having worked. I felt like I'd gotten some information, the eggs were good enough. Maybe it will work next time; I felt like we had a plan. I cried all weekend, and then I woke up Monday feeling pretty positive. I told people it hadn't worked. I said, "No it didn't work this time. We're going to do it again." I called my brother and I said, "Yeah, I've got to go back for that second test, it's part of the protocol, but I know I'm not pregnant, so whatever."

I felt I would know if I was. That's what I felt. I was so sure. I was so in tune with my body at this point. I was so aware of every little change. I had charted my temperature, my cervical position. You name it, I had charted it. I had done extensive research on fertility. If there's a book out there, I've read it. In the final analysis, I thought I was so in tune with my body that I would know.

I knew the nurse at this office very well. She said, "So where are you going to be later?" And I said, "I'll be at work, but just leave a message." She's like, "I'm not going to leave a message!" I said, "I know it's negative. Don't worry. I'm not going to be upset. I'm totally over it, it's fine."

It's because they knew I was pregnant.

And the reason she felt pretty sure with me is our levels were so high because we had *twins!* They felt pretty sure it couldn't have been a false positive. In fact they were pretty sure it was multiples just from the levels of hCG that kept tripling every time I went.

When they called . . . I had not given it another thought. I'm just going about my business. She's like, "You're pregnant." I really thought she was joking. And she said, "No, actually we don't joke about that. That would be bad."

And I had had all these fantasies about how I was going to tell my husband I was pregnant and everything. Forget it. I called him hysterically crying.

MICHAEL: I thought her mother had died, or somebody had just died.

ANNE: He wasn't the first to know. My colleague . . . I was crying so loudly that she didn't even knock, she burst into my office because she thought I had gotten a call that I wasn't pregnant. Who reacts like this if you are? I was so overwhelmed because I was so sure I wasn't. I was so surprised.

Alexandra had almost the same reaction. She prepared herself for the worst and for several days even experienced the worst, living in the failure that she anticipated.

ALEXANDRA: It was during Mardi Gras, and Peter got this baby in the king cake at work, and all these funny things were happening.

I was told after my transfer on Friday that I could have some cramping during the weekend, and that did not mean the transfer was being rejected. I should just breathe deeply and get through it and calm down. I had no cramps. I was so happy. I made it through an entire week. Nine days later, on Sunday, or ten days later, the following Sunday, I felt a little cramping. I was not happy about this because that would be exactly on day twenty-one of my cycle, and my blood test was scheduled for the following Friday, February 16, and I was beside myself. The cramps got worse on Monday and I was in a Greenspan hearing, I will never forget, and it was really bad. I called the nurse, Barbara, and she was like, umh, and I said they felt just like period cramps and she said, "any blood?" I said no and she goes, "Okay." She's like, "Just hang in there and let us know tomorrow."

That night I couldn't deal with it anymore, and I did the pregnancy test, which you are not supposed to do because you just get a false positive from the drugs. Well I wanted the false positive; I wanted it to get me to my blood test, so I did the pregnancy test at home. Negative.

Peter finds me bawling, and I'm like, "It didn't work."
He goes, "What do you mean?"

"I took the pregnancy test."

"You're not supposed to."

I said, "Peter, it's negative. There is no false positive. There is no false hope, there is no real hope. There is no hope."

PETER: It was so depressing. Later we found out that the hormones accelerate so quickly when it happens that had she done it twelve hours later, maybe it would've been positive.

ALEXANDRA: Or even in the morning, like eight hours later, you know? So anyway, unbelievable, it was so dark Monday night. So I go to work on Tuesday, and I am falling apart, and the cramps on the way home Tuesday night were even worse, and Peter says he still has hope, he got the little baby in the king cake, and I said, "You can have hope because you don't have a uterus, and you've never felt a period cramp. I know exactly what these are." Whoever has the most hormones wins, thank you very much, so I knew what I was feeling, and I was waiting for the blood.

PETER: Clearly you were right.

ALEXANDRA: I called the doctor's office, and literally the nurse was like, "This is bad."

The doctor's office offered to let Alexandra take the test early, the next day. She didn't sleep that night, worrying instead about telling her friends and family that the IVF hadn't worked.

ALEXANDRA: How do you call people and say, "I am losing a battle with fertility, and you might never be a grandparent, and I need to go to Russia and adopt a baby. I was turning it over in my mind that I was not pregnant. Totally. There was not an iota of hope in my body. I went in the next morning.

I was all choked up, like "Things aren't looking good for me," totally crying in front of the waiting room and in front of everybody. It was a nightmare.

I had the blood test and she is like, I will never forget it, she's like, "Just because you're cramping doesn't mean you aren't . . ."

I said, "You know what, thanks, but you have no idea what you're talking about."

I drove myself to Pentagon City Mall. I bought these high, strappy heels at Nine West and just wandered around. I was so crazed. I was just trying to keep myself busy, and I came back, and it was rainy. At ten of one I refused to answer the phone because it was Valentine's Day, and I knew my mother would call and be like, "Hi lovers! Happy Valentine's Day!"

I was lying in bed, and I had my little candle on, and I had all the lights out in the room, and it was dark and rainy, and I was in this saddest, sorriest state. I was writing in my journal like this was just the worst despair I have ever felt.

I just didn't know what to do. It was the end of the earth. I just felt like even though you can do in vitro again, it was so scary because it is the court of last resort. The clock really starts ticking. I felt like I was running out of options.

So I was bawling, and the phone rang and I didn't pick it up, and then I listen to the message and it was my doctor, and I thought, this is so sweet. This is why he makes big money, you know, when he really has to take you down off the cliff, he tells you instead of the nurse. I called right back and I said to the people, "Dr.—— just called me, and I just missed him. If he calls me back at home I will answer the phone this time."

Then I called Peter. Peter was supposed to take the day off, and then he couldn't, so he was trying to take a half day, and I said you have to come home, I am getting the bad news and he's like, "I can't come home right now."

PETER: I was very depressed at this point. I thought she shouldn't have taken the pregnancy test, and I still had hope because I don't have the hormones, and I just believe in what the doctor said.

ALEXANDRA: I remember I said, "When are you coming home, the doctor's going to call soon!" The curtain was going to go down, and he needed to be there, and he literally said something to the effect of, "You can cry when I get there."

I remember thinking I wasn't even mad at him. I thought Peter was just running out of things to say. This is one of those moments as a human being where you're just, the rubber meets the road.

The phone rang, and the doctor said, "How are you doing?"

I said, "I am hanging on, how are you?"

And he goes, "I am doing well. You are pregnant."

I just flipped out. I mean my heart started pounding. I said, "No, Doctor, I don't think they explained it to you." I was trying to tell him why I wasn't.

I said maybe they messed up the blood test, and he goes, "No, I remember what good quality embryos you had, and I am not supposed to tell you this, but for an early blood test, the numbers are so high, it looks like it might be twins."

I remember it was so physical a reaction, like my body was just tripping out. I can feel it right now. I was getting all tingly and cold. I am getting tingly now. I was just freaking out, literally physically freaking out. I was trying to fight back tears, and I was like, "Doctor, I can't thank you enough! We can't thank you enough!"

He was so sweet, he's like, "You just did," or he said something so adorable, and I remember so well that I could feel how much he was enjoying it.

PETER: I remember calling to find out what the status was and no one answering and then just saying I gotta get out of here, and just left.

ALEXANDRA: After all we went through, I was like, I am not telling him over the phone, I am just not telling him over the phone. He has got to show up here, and I will tell him in person. I got off the phone. I started crying and heaving and it was just this (screams) . . . like this relief! I can't explain it. I never experienced anything like it. It was so too good to be true. I was just charting this course from our French doors into the kitchen and into the living room over into the corner, and I kept pacing, and I was hyperventilating. I was like, I am probably going to give myself a miscarriage. I was going so crazy. I couldn't jump up and down, but it was so physical, it was like I had to keep moving, I had to keep moving, and I was just being taken over, and then you're like, 'I can't believe that I am really pregnant!' You know it's just so weird. But really it was that feeling like when you have a cancer test, and you think you have cancer, and you think you are going to die, and then they pull back from the brink. I mean it is just one of those pull-back-from-the-brink experiences where it is like—your worst fear is not true, and then not only is it not true, there is good news. It was such a combination!

So Peter walked in the house, and I was crying. I couldn't stop crying, and he walked in and he goes . . .

PETER: I thought it was bad news.

ALEXANDRA: He goes, "Awww," and I said, "We did it!" He was like, "Huh?"

I just could barely get the words out. I was like, "We did it!"

It was so weird because he couldn't even really get happy. He goes, "Oh my God, I knew there was hope!" But he wasn't really happy, he was kind of just relieved.

PETER: Well, yeah, I was happy, but it was very counterintuitive, I guess because, you know, I was really depressed, and I don't think I get depressed, regularly. I was anticipating the worst, and then when I came back—the mood in the house—she was just sitting there hunched over like, paralyzed, on a rainy day, like it was bad news, and so when she said, "We did it!" and she's crying, it took me a while to realize it was a party and not a funeral. But I was happy and excited. Definitely relieved.

ALEXANDRA: I remember vividly, I was too crazy. I couldn't even really get happy. I was just in my "It's over, the longing, the battle, it's over." I was in that mode. The shock. The relief and the shock.

I've thought long and hard about why success in IVF is so hard to fathom. All I can come up with is: time. Infertility is such a long, emotional, painful syndrome that when you come out of it, it just doesn't seem real. Your world becomes all about "No," and so a sudden, "Yes" just doesn't compute. It may be something like coming back from the brink of a deadly disease. You've lived your life for so long in one mindset, almost come to peace with it, and then suddenly everything you've thought about and experienced for years is no longer the reality.

IVF is also so scientific, so devoid of emotion, that such an emotional result is hard to accept. I think Tim and Kathy, who were also successful on the first try, said it best:

> KATHY: The steps make you, well they really have a foolproof system in the sense that you prepare yourself for anything. You prepare yourself almost not to be pregnant more than pregnant. You don't get your hopes up. We did not expect the first try to work.
>
> TIM: In the back of my mind, a friend of mine had had a miscarriage before . . . you had to wait three months. The whole time, with the steps of IVF and talking to the doctors and everything, I always tried in my mind to keep it as a clinical science project, that this is how we're looking at it, very clinically. This is a hassle, there are hurdles that we have to jump over; we don't have a baby yet.
>
> KATHY: You can never celebrate because you were always into the next phase.
>
> TIM: That way kept it emotionally low key for us because, as opposed to every time we cross this hurdle, excitement? No, let's not do that.

KATHY: The first ultrasound did it.

TIM: That's where it stopped being a science project for us, in the sense that we're now normal pregnant people!

"Normal" is a strong word for an IVF pregnancy, but, again, I'll get to that later. For me, there was and is nothing normal about having children through IVF. The emotions are unique to the procedure and therefore foreign to any hopes, dreams, or fantasies one may have had about getting pregnant.

There is, of course, joy, but it is a tempered joy at best. The incredulity, for me at least, totally overwhelmed the joy. I definitely felt a sense of relief and accomplishment, but when I think about how I found out, it was something of a letdown.

The older I get, the better I know that fantasies don't come true. Wishes may, but they never happen the way you hope they will. When I was little, I used to make my mother tell me over and over again about how she told my father she was pregnant with me. His answer was, "You're kidding!" It was a happy, natural, inevitable story that I'm sure replays itself over and over again in households all over the world.

Planned or unplanned, it is usually the woman who gets pregnancy news first; she gets to hold it all to herself for as long as she chooses, and then she gets to decide exactly how to tell her partner this cherished secret. With IVF, there is no secret. There are too many people and procedures involved. It is a cold, sterile, very public method of what should be a private, sensual, intimate act of love.

CHAPTER 10

TRY, TRY AGAIN

Anyone who's ever had twins has experienced the "blocker." Newborn babies often attract oglers, but the blocker is unique to twins. This is the person who will literally stand in front of your stroller, complimenting, questioning, admiring, and reminiscing, and completely blocking you from going on your merry way until they're good and ready to let you. Tiny twins are blocker magnets, and the questions are usually the same, as are my answers. Whenever they ask, "Are these your first?" I always say, "First and last!"

Maybe it's because I'm still in the toddler stage, maybe it's because I have a boy and a girl, but probably it's because I just can't imagine going through IVF again. I wonder if I would feel that way if we hadn't been successful. My guess is no.

Of the many people I spoke with who tried IVF multiple times, the issue of whether to try a second or third time usually involved only money. Other factors didn't come into play until the couple had gone through at least three unsuccessful cycles. The process, they said, was much easier the second time because they knew what to expect from the daily injections of drugs.

The 2001 CDC report on assisted reproductive technology found that in that year in America, IVF had a 25 percent success rate. These numbers, however, change depending on the factors of your infertility. For example, our doctor suggested that we would have a 50 percent chance of being successful because I was still young and the infertility was male factor. In other words, there is no way to give anyone an exact ratio, but suffice it to say that IVF fails more than it succeeds, and that means most couples will have to decide how many times to try. They all will have to find their limit.

I realize what I'm about to do is unfair, but it's my book, so I'll do it anyway. I'm going to introduce a new couple, right in the middle of everything. This couple tried IVF *five* times before it worked, with donor eggs on the last try. They had such a tremendously practical attitude and yet such an emotionally intense desire, I really found their thoughts quite remarkable.

Suffice it to say they are a couple of means who also had plenty of insurance coverage. I will call them simply "husband" and "wife."

WIFE: At every stage I kept thinking, I can't believe I am here, I can't believe I am letting them do this. I can't believe I opted to do this, but somehow it is incremental, and you sign up. If I had to sign up on the first day we went to see the doctor, and I was thirty-two or thirty-three, if I had to sign a form saying, "Yes, I will do five IVF cycles," there is no way I would have signed it, but after you do three IVF cycles, it seems kind of reasonable to do a fourth and after you do four, there was a big pause in terms of doing the fifth.

HUSBAND: I also think that because we had some help with insurance and because we were both working at good jobs, we didn't hit the end of our bank account, which I know has happened to other people. They simply can't afford to go on. Someone in my office who has now adopted two children said basically they looked at their finances and said we can either adopt or we can do IVF, but we can't do both, and one path will definitely lead us to a child, and one may not, so they decided to adopt. Fortunately we didn't have to make that decision, and maybe at some point we would've stopped for some other reason, but we weren't going to spend ourselves out of it.

This couple spent six years tied to IVF. There were successes, pregnancies, but they ended in miscarriage, and it wasn't like they could just jump right in over and over. Doctors will insist that a woman take some time off to recover after a miscarriage, and then of course there are the effects of all the drugs involved in IVF that you also need to take a break from. A lot of people don't realize that IVF is not just a six-week process. It takes physical as well as emotional recovery time, and that can translate into years of trying.

WIFE: You add the pregnancies, you add miscarriages, so let's say you get pregnant in January. Okay, let's say you are pregnant January, February, March, then you miscarry in April, they're not going to let you do anything again until maybe July. So then in the course of that year, you have the potential to do what? One IVF cycle? Two? I mean that is the thing I think people don't understand, but you can't just do one right after another.

Finally, after four tries, they decided to use donor eggs, which gave them hope but cost them even more time. It's not as if there are a bevy of women lined up to sell their eggs. You have to find the right person and then you have to find the right time. Again, more waiting.

> WIFE: It was probably a six-month setup. Then once we finally get in line, then it is a twelve-month wait. Then you have to wait for everybody's cycle to get in sync. It was practically two years, just doing that last cycle.

Imagine waiting and wanting for all that time! I knew that feeling for about a year, but I still can't imagine going through it for much more than that. I do, however, know of many others who waited even longer. It's not as if time flies when you're having fun, but time can really pass quickly when you are constantly looking toward deadlines, the next week, the next month. You spend so much time looking ahead that you don't even realize all the hours and days passing you by. Personally, I have no idea what we did during that year we were trying infertility treatments. Nothing stands out. For a lot of couples, it is time spent at home, doing nothing because socializing is often too difficult. Everyone around you seems to either have or be having kids, and even that standard dinner-table conversation of "What's new?" becomes too daunting to face. We really shut out the world, and many others in our situation do too.

HUSBAND: There really wasn't much else going on. I mean that really was the single, dominant fact about my life, and I am sure my wife's too, through that whole time . . . you know, we are trying to get pregnant.

WIFE: At some point when you do IVF, you realize, you know, I can do this for the next twenty years. It's stressful, but it's not like you spend hours a day doing IVF. You don't. Yeah, you've got to find a bathroom to do your injections, but you are out of the bathroom in ten minutes, so it's not like you can't go to work. It was stressful in terms of getting it to work out with my job, but I did go to work, and I worked a lot of hours, and I worked hard, and I got promotions, and it's not like it kept us from going out and socializing. We just structured things a little differently. It's not like it even kept us from going on vacation. Granted I look at our vacation pictures and our vacation pictures are all kind of sad-looking people because we always went on vacations after miscarriages when we knew, okay we are timed out here for two months, we might as well go on a vacation.

Also we were having some successes in there. Obviously they weren't successful pregnancies that went to term, but if we did get pregnant on two or three IVF cycles, the idea of doing a fourth one doesn't seem like such a wacky idea, or it doesn't seem like such an impossible thing to contemplate.

But after a while, it did seem less and less practical to keep doing the same thing, and that's when they turned to donor eggs. For the wife, this was obviously not an easy decision; she was giving up the possibility of passing on her genetic code, not to mention the fact that she was going to actually carry someone else's child. But like couples who choose to adopt, she realized that being a mother was more important to her than genetics. This was really her last option other than adoption.

> WIFE: Well at that point, I was simply getting old. At every IVF cycle (we had a cycle where we didn't even get to retrieval) I became less and less responsive to the medicines. I talked to someone in the donor egg program, and she said that of the eight people, I mean this is a very small sample, but of the eight people they had with recurrent miscarriages, those who had been lucky enough to conceive with donor eggs all made it to term. Both of us thought that if the heart of this is maybe some kind of immunology problem, and maybe there is just something about the two of us that is never going to work together genetically, it seemed like the last kind of option. The plan was we would officially put this all to bed. It was the very last thing we were going to do.

Still, again, this was as great a leap for the wife as was trying IVF in the first place.

> HUSBAND: I think it was less of a leap for me because I was not giving up my genetic connection to our future child, and I thought it really was the only realistic chance we had,

given our difficulties in conceiving and then recurrent miscarriages; I really thought that there was some sort of hormonal or immunological problem that resulted from the combination, and we had some medical reason to think that that might be going on, although nobody really wanted to say for sure. For me, I thought that this is a change we can make that will improve our chances, but I think probably my wife felt differently about it.

WIFE: It is a very complicated thing. In a way I felt very secure. I felt like, okay, well maybe the problem has always been my eggs, and now I have eggs from somebody who has had a child, now I have eggs from someone whose numbers are just phenomenal. So for me, there was a sense of security.

I absolutely did not want to be pregnant again with my own eggs, and I didn't want to do another IVF cycle. Still, my husband was much more into doing the donor egg cycle than I was, in large part because I didn't want to get pregnant again. I really was fearful about being pregnant and did not want to have to go through being pregnant again.

But they did, and finally it worked. They were finally going to be parents. They said that if it hadn't worked that time, with the donor eggs, they probably would have given up. That was their limit. That was all they could do.

CHAPTER 11

NO

W e always said three tries would be our limit with IVF. Was that a lie? How could we ever know when enough would really be enough? I look at my children now, and think that I would have done IVF a hundred times if someone could have guaranteed me that this would someday be the result. But as I've said over and over, in IVF there are no guarantees. Even the big fertility clinics that offer the money-back guarantees give up at three or four tries. The fact is, if you haven't gotten pregnant after that many, the odds are you probably won't at all.

So how do you give up? How do you come to terms with the fact that you will never have a genetic child of your own? Some, like the couple in the last chapter, will opt for donor eggs or donor sperm, getting at least half a genetic match. Others will use surrogates to carry their own embryos or a mix and match. There are options, but they are expensive and can ultimately end in the same disappointment, and the couple will have to face the same question: when do you give up?

Carol and Mike spent ten years and $75,000 battling infertility. They tried drugs, operations, and three cycles of IVF. When they began, Carol was thirty years old. She was over forty when they finally threw in the towel. What made them say no? They said money. They have a dual annual income of less than $100,000, and it was only because they came into some money from a friend's will that they were able to try as many procedures as they did. But in talking to them at length, I could see that it was more than just money. Their hope and their marriage were both on shaky ground. Both had had invasive medical procedures and they were just plain tired. Their lives had been so wrapped up in this battle for so long that they seemed to have lost touch with their own relationship. They poured their souls into a family that just wouldn't materialize, and in doing so they came close to losing the foundation of that family, their own bond with each other. Mike says he's not sure they ever really recovered. Maybe not, but they finally did move on.

> MIKE: In my dreams I just got up and walked out of the fertility clinic, but I didn't really. I said thank you very much, we'll talk to you. And we did come home, and we had some very tearful conversations . . . do we go back? Do we try it one more time? Or do we take this money and just go get some kids? After talking about it for about a week or so, we said, we've had the roller-coaster, let's go see what we can do on adoption.

What still eats at both of them, though, is the feeling that they missed the boat, that had they been just a little bit younger, started just a few years earlier, they would have had a legitimate chance. At that time, the science was still evolving, the techniques were changing and improving with every year.

Recovering from a decade of trying was also not an easy task. Mike had an easier time of it than Carol. Before his surgery to remove epididymal sperm, he had thought he would never be a biological father. They had already used donor sperm more than once, so he was at peace with that.

> MIKE: From my point of view, I'd gotten over the grieving process because it had been decided years before that I was not going to be able to be a biological father. So then when all of a sudden I had sperm that was viable and could be used, that was like a blessing. But I had already gone through the grieving process of not being able to be a biological father. I don't think I went through it again.
>
> But for Carol, even after we made the decision, no more, it was a good six months back to reasonable physical shape and emotional shape.
>
> CAROL: I don't know that I would really say I was depressed that much, just angry at everything that had gone on, everything that I'd been through, the feelings that nobody really cared, and I just had to go on and focus on something else and find a way to just get past it.
>
> MIKE: I think that the one thing that kept her from feeding into any type of a depression, either from the drugs or from the fact that we'd gone through all this and it didn't work, was we immediately moved into the adoption process, and that was such a busy process of getting all the papers, getting all the home visits done, getting everything done that had to get done that there really wasn't time to focus on the failures.

CAROL: The first visit that we made to [the adoption agency] to make inquiries into adoption was March of that year. A couple of months max . . . maybe a month and a half after we gave up. We'd been grieving for a long time, because it hadn't been working, so it was just time to say okay.

Carol and Mike adopted a boy and a girl, who are not related, but look surprisingly alike and remarkably like them. The boy had actually been abandoned, left on the streets of a remote Russian city, left to die. The children are well aware of where they came from. They proudly showed me pictures of themselves as babies in Russia. They have Russian dolls and toys in their Virginia home; their culture feels like another member of the family, and a cherished one at that.

You could say that this is a sad story mixed with a happy ending, but it is far more complicated than that. Carol and Mike clearly adore their children, but it's not hard to see the disappointment they still feel when talking about their battle with infertility.

MIKE: I remember the first time we got pregnant through IVF. The technician gave me an ultrasound picture and said, "Here's your first birthday picture of your kids!" I carried that around for a week, until she lost the embryos. I thought, it's gonna work, and then you're back to square one. And Carol would say, "I need to take some time." Especially after the first one. She was so devastated, physically, that we waited a couple of months before we tried again.

The emotions today are as clear in his memory as they were more than a decade ago. When I met them, they had already been

parents for several years, but they talked about their fight with infertility as if it were just yesterday.

Giving up just one more try was probably one of the hardest
things either of them will ever have to do. That's the way IVF works,
even when it doesn't work. Because it is the last resort for so many
people, it just seems like it has to keep doling out hope. To this day,
Carol still doesn't know exactly what kept her from conceiving a
child, and perhaps that's why the IVF hope was so hard to let go. She
spent a decade living with IVF's unique brand of hope and then with
its ensuing, devastating failure. Where did a decade go? Neither she
nor Mike can really remember, but it went. The experience will always be part of their lives.

For Chris and Kate, the ordeal was faster, but it was equally
painful in the end. Their first reaction was that maybe they had done
something wrong, not the science, but them. It's amazing how careful
and exact you feel you have to be when doing IVF. I guess it's because
there is so much at stake, but no normal pregnant person, I don't care
how cautious, acts like a person trying to get pregnant from IVF.
People get pregnant all the time, often in nonideal situations. I doubt
the average woman thinks about her eggs every month, worries about
where they're sitting in her body and, in turn, in which direction she
should sit while watching TV or even going to the bathroom. But for
an IVF mother, every second of that time when the embryo has been
implanted and is waiting to take or not, directions, positions, actions,
and nerves are topic A. Kate was no exception, as she describes her
emotions after the fertilized eggs were transferred to her uterus.

KATE: So they told me I had to drink a lot of water, which
I did, and then I'm lying there on the table, and they tell me

I didn't drink enough water, and I'm like, "You don't understand, I'm in so much pain right now, I have to pee so bad," and they're like, "That's the tiniest bladder I have ever seen."

So they do the transfer, which is a little bit uncomfortable, and I lay on the table for I think like thirty minutes in the other room, and then we get up and go home. I had taken the whole week off. I was a little worried. I lied on the couch. And they only tell you, just go easy. They say don't lift anything, don't vacuum . . . you don't need to lie on the couch for five days, but you need to take it easy. I said, okay, I'm taking the whole week off from work.

For the first three days I laid down as much as possible. I wish I had been more of a freak about it. I was excited, wow, these are embryos, these are my children inside me and I want them to stay there, so I made Chris carry me up the stairs. My mother said, "You make Christopher carry you, don't you walk up those stairs!"

You're so worried, oh my gosh, are they implanting? Are they still there? Are they doing what they need to do? Am I resting enough? I was worried the whole time.

CHRIS: I had taken off some time from work and came up with the bright idea of putting Kate in the car and driving two and a half hours to my parents' place at the beach just north of Jacksonville. I sold it to Kate as, you can sit in a chaise lounge on the deck and relax at the oceanside. So we did that and we had a chance to visit with my folks and we drove back two days later. I often wonder if maybe that wasn't a good idea.

KATE: Maybe I should have just lay in bed for five days . . .
CHRIS: Not that she did anything too strenuous, but five hours in the car, the constant vibration, I don't know.

In all my research I never found anything that showed one way or the other that staying in bed or trying not to move made any difference at all in the success of IVF. Think about it: most women who aren't doing IVF, whether they're trying to get pregnant or not, rarely know the exact day that their fertilized embryo reaches their uterus. This knowledge is unique to the IVF patient. Yes, when you're trying to get pregnant naturally, doctors might tell you to put your legs up or lie on your back for half an hour after sex (how many times I did this!), but that's just to help the semen stay in the body and to give the sperm the benefit of gravity to get to their goal.

During IVF, the embryo is shot up through the vagina with a catheter and actually "placed" in the uterus. It would really have no more chance of "falling out" than any other embryo that enters the uterus naturally by way of the fallopian tube. I honestly think doctors tell women to lie down and relax because stress plays a huge factor with anyone trying to get pregnant. Relaxing and letting the body rest is beneficial of course, but it's not like you do it to keep the embryo in place.

KATE: On the day we were to find out, I had a field trip. I went into the doctor's office before work and I was so worried about finding out, I made Chris go on the field trip with me.
CHRIS: Really, we debated whether or not she should even go to work that day, but we figured we were going to be finding out one way or another . . . We went to the field trip and . . .

CHRIS: Got the call.

KATE: We got the call. It was the nurse and she said, well, as soon as she said my name, I could tell. She said, "Kate," I said, "Yeah." "I have some news and it's not good." And after that honestly I can't remember what the words were, it was just that I wasn't pregnant. It didn't work.

CHRIS: She broke into tears on the phone.

KATE: I had to let my aide take the kids.

CHRIS: Turns out that wasn't such a good idea going to work that day. Kate and I took a nice little walk to the other side of the park and had a good cry.

KATE: I made him ride home on the bus with me. I mean, I don't know why. I probably could have just left, but we got on the bus and we went back to school and then I called my mother. I told her I didn't want to have to tell anybody else so could she take care of that for me. She said, "Okay, I'm so sorry, of course I'll do that for you."

So we went back to work and I told my three friends that knew I was waiting to find out. I told them and then I told my principal and asked if I could leave, and we got in my car and we came home.

I think I just cried and . . . it was just really sad and so disappointing that it didn't work and we pretty much decided we weren't going to do it again. I didn't want to have to go through the pain and all of that again. I was tired of being disappointed. This was like three years of trying to get pregnant. The constant disappointment of not being pregnant . . .

CHRIS: It was running our lives.

KATE: It was running our lives and it was just too much. I was so depressed and unhappy and I felt like I wasn't myself anymore. I was just really tired of trying to get pregnant. It really just was consuming our lives and I wasn't happy.

CHRIS: For me it was the hand we were dealt, and it was a bitter pill to swallow but it was also okay. Here you are, this is what you've got, and what are you going to do about it? When Kate's depressed or upset, that's . . . my main goal is to try to pick up a little bit. I just felt so bad about how things went not only for myself but I really felt bad for Kate because I knew what she went through, and at that point in time it just opened the door for us for adoption. I said, you know what, you want to do something, we could adopt, and this is where we're supposed to go.

KATE: Almost instantly okay, that's it, we've done IVF, we've tried, this is not what is supposed to be happening for us, there must be a baby out there in the world already waiting for us because for us to have our own is just really not meant to be. We did consider IVF again, we really did, and we talked about it again, briefly.

CHRIS: I remember that conversation and I remember my feelings at that point in time were it's just the end of the infertility chapter of our lives. It was done. It was the emotional angle. I wasn't ready for Kate to go through this all again.

KATE: It would have been do IVF, come up with thirty grand, or come up with thirty grand for adoption, and at that time I was just over it. Of course I wanted to be pregnant and have my own baby, but this was too much. I couldn't handle it anymore. I just couldn't tell people anymore that here I am, I'm not pregnant. It didn't happen. I wasn't just over it.

CHRIS: And you know that people feel sorry for you and you just don't want to dwell in this depressed state all the time and you reach a point where you say no. We could not have children and still be happy with each other.

Chris and Kate adopted a beautiful little boy from Russia. His name is Noah.

Most couples will try IVF for years and years before turning to adoption. The desire to have a biological child is that strong. In speaking to those who were unsuccessful at IVF, I found that the need doesn't come from wanting to be a parent. Anyone can be a parent to any child. It's more about the possibility to reproduce one's self. Some consider it a gift, others a right, but when people are stripped of the gift or the right, they usually feel that some judgment has been made about who they are. Somehow, someone has decided that they are not good enough to pass themselves on to another generation, that they are not worthy of finding immortality through their children.

And then of course there is the desire to be pregnant. So many women I've met who did not have fertility problems absolutely loved being pregnant. Yes, it's physically uncomfortable, and of course morning sickness isn't fun, but to spend nine months knowing that you are growing something inside you is really an incomparable experience. The rush of hormones, the excitement of feeling that life kicking in your belly, the almost star quality a pregnant woman elicits from family, friends, strangers in the supermarket. "Do you know what you're having?" "When are you due?" A pregnant woman is always the center of attention. All these traits are enviable to say the least and, if not the overall driving factor of motherhood, are certainly part of a woman's thought process when she considers having a baby. Not so for the adoptive mother.

The worst part of finite infertility is that there is no appeals process. There is nothing you can do, say, eat, or improve that will change the judgment that has been made upon you; it is final. You will not reproduce yourself genetically; your physical traits, your personality quirks, that look you get when you don't understand something, all of it, everything that lives naturally within you, will live and die with you. This is a demoralizing blow from which some people never truly recover. It is as if someone died, someone who was never even born.

YOUR PREGNANCY

CHAPTER 12

THIRTY-TWO WEEKS
AND TWO DAYS

As I said, some women just love being pregnant. I'd like to know what they're smoking. From start to finish, my pregnancy was just about the worst experience of my life. As much as I couldn't believe I was pregnant at first, I couldn't really accept being pregnant either. I never did. The sterile medical environment in which my children were conceived stole something from the natural emotions I had always expected to feel from pregnancy. Here was something I actively pursued for years, thought about constantly, daydreamed about on an hourly basis, and when I finally got there, it was as if I entered a room that didn't exist.

I realize that there are plenty of women who didn't do IVF who felt exactly as I did during pregnancy. There are plenty of non-IVFers who have harrowing pregnancies, end up on bed rest, miscarry early or late in the game, and who, even during flawless pregnancies, find themselves feeling angry, depressed, fearful, and deceived. There are as many experiences of pregnancy as there are pregnant women, and I don't mean to belittle those experiences by sharing my own. I also don't mean to say that I regret any moment of what I went through. I regret that I had a bad pregnancy; I don't regret that I got pregnant. It was and is the most important thing I have ever done in my life, and as many infertile couples will agree, it is a victory unlike any other.

I tell the story of my pregnancy in detail because I do believe that from day one my particular emotions were the result of IVF. I also believe that the stress and anguish of infertility and the resulting unnatural medical procedure colored my perspective on pregnancy and kept me from even the possibility of "normal" emotions. And I know I'm not alone.

More than a year after my initial interview with Anne and Michael, I called Anne for a follow-up chat. She and Michael had been pretty clear during our first interview that they were a little more than reluctant to have any more children after the birth of their twins. When we spoke the second time, the twins were already four years old, and Anne confided in me that she had recently been considering trying to get pregnant. After much soul-searching, however, she decided not to. Her reasoning was eerily familiar to me. She said that when she really examined her desire to have another child, she discovered that what she really wanted was to have a normal pregnancy. She wanted another shot at that exciting time in so many women's lives that she had missed out on because of her battle with infertility and her doing IVF. She had watched so many of her friends enjoy not only their pregnancies but those first months of infancy, and she had a strong envy inside her.

Anne went over and over her possible scenarios in her mind. She knew she would probably have to go through IVF again, and even if it were a single pregnancy and not twins, she finally admitted to herself that no IVF pregnancy was going to be normal. In any case, she thought, the desire to experience a happy pregnancy was no reason to have a child. But it was strong enough to make her consider it seriously. This is why I tell my story.

Day one, I'm excited, nervous, thrilled, calling the family and telling the news. By day two I'm sure I'm going to have a miscarriage. For some reason, most likely the IVF reason, I felt that *staying* pregnant was going to be just as hard as *getting* pregnant. I read the statistics about the number of pregnancies that end in miscarriage, and I was sure that I would fall into that category; after all, the chances of being infertile were much smaller than the chances of miscarriage, and I managed to make that cut.

And then there was the waiting, more waiting, almost constant waiting. Unlike a normal pregnancy, IVF is a series of closely monitored tests. First you have to find out if you're actually pregnant, that is, if the embryos attached to your uterus and signaled the appropriate hormones to begin growth. I had already waited the two weeks after the transfer to find that out. But there's more. Since most IVFs involve multiple embryo transfer, you have to wait another four weeks, the period in which the embryos become large enough to see on sonogram, to find out exactly how many are in there and if they in fact have heartbeats. Again, when a regular, fertile couple finds out they're pregnant, that's about it for quite a while. They just wait to get big. Most don't have the first sonogram until they are already twenty weeks along. To me, those four weeks were one grand bout of PMS. The drugs left me so bloated and crampy that I was sure every time I pulled down my pants I would see red. It is also quite common to spot a little bit during the first weeks of pregnancy, and I did. To me, this was yet another sign of trouble.

I also felt fragile. Because this pregnancy was not exactly natural, in my mind I somehow felt like it was less, well, binding than a normal pregnancy. I imagined that because the embryo had not traveled a normal path to get to my uterus it was more likely to fall out. Granted, every one of these thoughts is irrational. Nevertheless, I was thinking them day and night.

Finally, after what seemed like the longest four weeks of my life, we went back to Dr. Sacks for our first sonogram. Because this first one is done so early in the pregnancy, it has to be done internally. I had had plenty of internal sonograms during the previous months. It's often done during IUI to make sure the uterus is ready, and it is done during the IVF for retrieval as well as transfer. This time, however, was different. That long mechanical probe may have been heading for the same area, but this time there were occupants, and I was terrified the device would knock them out. Again, irrational, but what do I know?

So there I am, lying in my favorite position, knees in the air, uterus on the air, or on the little monitor at least, waiting for the verdict. Slowly and carefully, Dr. Sacks moved the probe into position and pointed at the screen to what looked like a tiny, pulsing, gray swish.

"There it is," he said, in his usual calm demeanor. There was life. Okay, it's there, we're all right. For a few minutes, at least, we're still pregnant. Before I could even breathe a tiny sigh of relief (not that I could ever really breathe with that thing stuck up me) Dr. Sacks was talking again.

"Okay, now panning down to the left here, there's the other one."

Excuse me?

The other one.

Twins. Obviously we knew this was a possibility. We put two embryos back in, and Scott, in his usual optimistic vein, was sure we'd get twins. But I wasn't. I couldn't even believe in one, let alone two. But there they were, two gray swishes. The nurse, the one who had told me weeks before that I was "knocked up," grabbed my hand and asked if I was okay. I didn't know.

When I asked friends of mine what it was like when they first found out they were pregnant, they described feelings of warmth and joy and wafting love toward their husbands. They talked about sensing life inside them and suddenly getting their first real sense of motherhood, of responsibility over something growing inside them. I got none of that.

Those two swishes on the screen were a complete disconnect. The problem was, everything about my children's conception was a disconnect. Remember, I was twelve blocks away when they were conceived. I guess I shouldn't have been surprised that I would have a hard time picturing them as a part of me. Most women learn of their pregnancies through their own bodies. They either miss a period or watch their own pee turn a stick a different color. Everything about my pregnancy, I saw on a TV monitor. Ironic, I know. This was the one time I didn't want to be on TV.

We left the office with our first pictures. Gray swishes on glossy rolled-up paper. This was my pregnancy. Scott and I went across the street to a little bakery and shared a muffin. We stared at each other, not knowing really what to say. Everything we had done had worked, all of it. One dose of IVF, and we were pregnant with twins. All at once we felt like the luckiest people on earth, but, for me at least, unsure as to what I had just won. It just didn't seem real, probably because it had taken so long to achieve.

It wasn't the twins. It seems so strange to me now, but when I was pregnant, from that day in the little bakery forward, I never really thought much about twins. This is something I deeply regret because only now do I know how completely uninformed I was. Multiple pregnancies are high risk, and while knowing this would not have changed our decision to transfer two embryos, more information on twin pregnancies would definitely have helped me prepare for what was ahead. The trouble is, when you're infertile and embarking on IVF, you are so wrapped up with the getting there that you often don't anticipate the being there. IVF is information overload and often, as many of the couples I spoke with agreed, you spend so much time learning about IVF that you don't learn about pregnancy and especially multiple pregnancy, which is the result of one-third of all IVFs.

I knew that with multiples there was a possibility of one surviving and one not. There is also something called a "phantom" pregnancy in which a second embryo is spotted on the sonogram, but it never develops a heartbeat. That was about all I knew, because to me that was still a part of the getting pregnant process.

Mine was definitely real twins. Two little people were preparing to enter my life, while one person was about to leave it. Dr. Sacks's work was done. He had accomplished exactly what we asked of him, and it was time for us to move on to a regular ob for a regular pregnancy. Right from the start he had told us that he makes babies, he doesn't do babies. Leaving him was harder than I anticipated. We had already come so far, but we had such a long way to go. I hated the fact that we had to trust this pregnancy, this masterful, long-awaited achievement, to anyone other than him. It just didn't seem right.

I know it's not at all uncommon for women to become attached to their obstetricians but the attachment to a fertility specialist runs deeper. With a normal ob, she may be responsible for getting you through the pregnancy, but you were the one who got yourself pregnant. With a specialist, you yourself have little sense of achievement in the pregnancy, or at least I didn't. I felt it was all him, so leaving him, without that trust in myself, was beyond disconcerting. Obviously I wasn't going back to my old ob, the one who had brushed me off so precipitously. Dr. Sacks recommended a nearby practice, and told me I would be in good hands, but I still didn't want to leave him, and even worse, I didn't know how to say goodbye. I'm sure this happens a lot with patients who have been cured of some terrible disease or survived a horrific accident. They see their doctors as close to gods. Dr. Sacks didn't save my life, but he did give me life—two lives. I came to him empty, and he filled out my future. "Thank you" seemed like a silly thing to say.

So we just left. He told us to keep in touch. We shook hands. It was strange. It was uncomfortable. For so many months I had felt so close to him, but now we had no reason to see each other. I hoped that one day we would come back and add a picture of our kids to his wall of fertile fame. I fantasized about it, but it seemed like such a long way away. So we just left.

There I was, pregnant with twins, a normal pregnant woman. According to science, I was no longer to consider this a special pregnancy, although twins made it high risk. IVF was simply a way to get there, and now it was over. There is no data to show that an IVF pregnancy acts any differently than a normal pregnancy. So why did it still feel so unnatural? Why couldn't I just feel pregnant?

Morning sickness would do it, I was sure. As soon as I threw up, I knew it would all fall into place. As soon as I threw up. I never threw up. About two months into the pregnancy, I began to feel queasy in the afternoons. My sense of smell was more sensitive than it had been, and there were certain things I just couldn't eat, like tomato sauce. But I never threw up, never even came close. There must be something wrong.

Okay, I know it says in the books that not every woman gets morning sickness, but I just wanted *something* in this pregnancy to be regular. I wanted a glow, a craving, a sign that I was just like every other woman going through the first months of pregnancy. I knew I shouldn't expect to be showing that early, but nothing was even tight. In fact, I lost some weight in the beginning, which, again, is not uncommon, but which to me was a sure sign that something was wrong.

I went to my new ob, expecting to get bad news, but when she put the little transistor radiolike thing up against my still-flat stomach, I heard the whooshing pulses of the heartbeats. They were still there, toying with my flaring emotions, prodding me to believe but not yet convincing me of their inherent truth. Even if they were in there, I was sure there was something wrong with them. The amnio would show it. We'd have to wait again to get the bad news.

Why were we doing amnio? Because I'm a freak. Amniocentesis is recommended for pregnant women over the age of thirty-five to detect genetic disorders like Down's syndrome. I was only thirty-four at the time, but my due date was three days after my thirty-fifth birthday. That meant that my health insurance would cover the procedure, so my new ob suggested we do it. I wanted to do it regardless because, despite all evidence to the contrary, I was sure that IVF would make us more prone to genetic disorders. I was sure that because this was not a natural pregnancy, more than likely the genetic codes didn't line up in the right order.

I also, frankly, wanted to know what we were having. I desperately wanted a boy and a girl, so there would be no reason to go through all this again. I knew that if we had two of the same that I would want to have another. Amnio, I was sure, would clear my mind of all fears and give me a real sense of pregnancy by knowing exactly what I was getting. This would be it. This would finally make me feel pregnant. This was a nightmare.

We waited until week fourteen, as is recommended, and went in for the test, but first you have to do this whole genetic counseling session, where they basically map out your medical family tree, each leaf a genetic malfunction. We had to sit there for about two hours telling the counselor about the aunt who died of breast cancer, the uncle who had multiple sclerosis, the cousin with Down's syndrome, and so on. By the time we left, we were both convinced our children were swimming not in amniotic fluid, but in a genetic cesspool.

The procedure itself was doubly awful. Basically, a large needle is inserted through the uterine wall into the amniotic sac, and fluid is withdrawn. The fluid carries the DNA of the baby and therefore can give you a pretty good idea of what you're getting. There is a risk with amnio of miscarriage, and of course that risk goes up if you have twins. Every amnio carries risk, but for an IVF mother, that risk is inflated, if not physically, emotionally. Again, any risk to the pregnancy means going back to the great infertility drawing board. I certainly don't mean to downplay the fact that plenty of normally conceived pregnancies miscarry, but when you've gone through IVF, it seems there is just so much more at stake, emotionally, physically, financially.

I asked the genetic specialist if she had ever lost a set of twins. In her twenty years, she said, she had lost one set, but, she assured me, that was because the woman's cervix (basically the doorway the baby eventually goes through to exit the uterus) had given way too early, and they couldn't save the pregnancy. It may or may not have had something to do with the amnio, but no one could ever know conclusively. Right then and there I made a mental note to have my cervix checked at every checkup.

Unfortunately, because a twin amnio is more complicated, the procedure was not as easy and painless as some had described. The doctor had a little trouble getting to both sacs and had to go in with the needle twice. I left the office furious at the added, unnecessary trauma and sure that I would miscarry. Surely the stress of all this was going to end the pregnancy. After all the needles I'd gone through to get there, that last needle was going to end it all. Amnio was supposed to make me feel more pregnant, I thought, and it did just the opposite.

Again, we waited. For two years we waited to get pregnant, for six weeks we waited through IVF, for two more weeks we waited for results, for six more weeks we waited to see if there were heartbeats, for six more weeks we waited for amnio, and now we had two weeks to wait for the results. When were we just going to be pregnant?

The results were supposed to take twelve to fourteen days, but on day ten I got a nice surprise. In yet another surreal phone call, the genetic counselor from our specialist's office called to say that everything looked great. There was no Down's syndrome or any other kind of genetic disorder they could see. And I was carrying a boy and a girl. Everything was perfect. Now, I thought, I could really be pregnant. Now the feeling would surely come.

About a week later, still stewing in the warm comfort of our amnio results, I walked into my office one morning to see the little red message light blinking on my phone. It was a nurse from my new ob's office. "We have the results of one of your blood tests. You need to call us immediately."

The little red message light turned off, just as I turned white. Something was wrong. After sitting on hold for several, interminable minutes, the nurse came on and, very matter-of-factly, informed me that I had tested positive for Gaucher's disease. What's Gaucher's disease? Who the *hell* knows? It was one of the many diseases listed when you take all those blood tests at the beginning of your pregnancy. I knew already that I was a carrier for Tay-Sachs, what they call a Jewish disease, but since Scott was negative, we were fine. I had never even heard of Gaucher's disease, that is, until the nurse spent fifteen minutes scaring me senseless. She told me that a baby born with Gaucher's disease would be horribly malformed and completely retarded and wouldn't live past six months. The chances of a person carrying Gaucher's were less than 5 percent, but apparently, once again, I had made the cut. She told me that if Scott was a carrier, like me, we had a fifty-fifty chance of each baby being born with it. I immediately got on the phone with the genetic specialist. She wanted to see the results and then see us in her office that evening.

From nine in the morning when I returned that message from the nurse to that five o'clock appointment with the specialist, my children were going to be born with a debilitating and deadly disease. My happy pregnancy of one week (since the amnio) was now over. I scoured the Internet and spun myself deeper and deeper into a despair spiral.

Scott and I arrived at the specialist's office a little before five, expecting to hear the very worst. Since we were an add-on emergency, we had to wait more than an hour. Finally, at six o'clock, we were ushered back into her little office. The first thing she told us to do was calm down. Calm down? Impossible.

It took some explaining, but apparently the nurse at the ob's had jumped to an incorrect conclusion. It seems there are three different kinds of Gaucher's. Two are terrible, one is not. I tested positive as a carrier for the one that is not. This form of Gaucher's, which is prevalent in the Jewish population (aren't we supposed to be the *Chosen* people?), is a minor liver disorder that may or may not even make itself known to the person who has it. A person could live a happy full life with even the worst case of it. If Scott had it, we would just have to be on the lookout as our babies grew up, but if he didn't, then there was no way the babies could have it.

Strangely enough, though, the specialist suggested we not even test Scott. She said that because of some ridiculous insurance complication that I refuse to get into, Scott could end up paying higher rates if he tested positive. We were fine, she assured us, just fine. Our babies would be fine. Go ahead, feel pregnant, I said to myself, but I knew it would take time again, time to recover. I still wasn't there.

Just as we were ready to go home and fantasize about the martini that I desperately needed but definitely couldn't have, the specialist noticed something in my chart. We hadn't been tested for cystic fibrosis. I didn't know we had to be tested for cystic fibrosis. Well, she said, it's a new test, and you might want to know. Scott and I looked at each other with the same battle-weary stare and said a collective "No." After the Gaucher's day we had just had, we said, "No more." Enough. Let the chips fall where they may. We were outta there.

Now it was time to be pregnant. Now I was ready to really enjoy it, feel it, experience it like everybody else. I had my sixteen-week checkup scheduled for the next week. I was beginning to show a little bit. Everything was going to be great.

And the checkup was fine. I insisted the doctor check my cervix, which she did, and all was holding up and in well. The heartbeats were strong, and my uterus was growing at a nice pace. Just as I was leaving, though, the doctor mentioned that she did not see a cystic fibrosis test result. I told her we decided not to do it. She asked why, and I couldn't really give her a good reason, other than that we were sick of doing genetic tests. She suggested that it really wasn't a big deal, just another vial of blood, and it really was important. Scott wasn't there, and for some reason I just said, okay, whatever, and went to have my blood drawn. She said the results would take a week. Fine.

It was December, and it was time for the big change I had been planning for months; this could also be the real beginning of my fantasy pregnancy. After seven years, I left my job at CBS and began work on this book. My plan was in motion. I would conduct my interviews at a leisurely pace, do my research from my dining room table, and swim laps at my nearby gym—a low-key, healthy, stress-free pregnancy was curtain up! This was the time, I thought, now I was really going to feel pregnant. We would start planning the nursery. I even allowed myself to buy a book of names and spent a little too much time surfing designer baby Web sites. We also went away for the holidays to visit both our families in New York and Boston, and I let my mother buy me some even bigger maternity clothes and schlep me through some baby furniture stores. I was letting myself see it. I really was. With everything going on, I forgot about all the tests, all the genetic silliness we had put ourselves through. We laughed about it. We were so neurotic.

When we got back from vacation, we had our twenty-week sonogram; that's the one where they can really see all the internal organs. Everything looked great. We even got this really funny picture of our little boy's not-so-little male material. I glimpsed joy. It was right outside the door that my anxiety-ridden psyche had slammed shut for so long. It was seeping through the cracks, seeping through my crackpot brain.

Until, of course, the ob's office called again. After a major delay of more than a month due to some freak snowstorm in the South where the genetic laboratory they use happens to be, the cystic fibrosis test results were back. I tested positive as a carrier—and this one isn't even prevalent among Jews! Again, as usual, my mind went reeling back to IVF. Was there a connection? I knew that our infertility problem was male factor, but something in my mind said that maybe it was me too. Maybe I didn't get pregnant because my body, carrying these awful diseases, was not supposed to reproduce. Nature was trying to protect a future unborn child from cystic fibrosis, and I selfishly intervened. Obviously, looking back, none of this makes any medical sense, but at the time it made plenty of sense to me.

Scott, of course, hadn't been tested, because we declined that day at the specialist's office. In yet another panic, that afternoon, he rushed back to see her and give blood. If he was a carrier, which he apparently had a 3 to 5 percent chance of being, then each of our babies had a 25 percent chance of getting it. Cystic fibrosis. This one I had heard of.

The results would take another week. Another week we would have to wait. I didn't sleep at all the first night. I sat at the computer at three in the morning, scouring the Internet for information on CF. The more I read, the more I was convinced that I would be spending the next twenty years shuttling my emaciated, wheezing twins back and forth from the hospital. I was so angry, angry that the tests had taken so long and that we were now well past the twenty-week mark. Not that I could imagine doing it, but at that point I didn't even have the option of ending the pregnancy. In my mind, for the umpteenth time, it was over. I actually threw out a stack of baby catalogs. I shut the door tight again on any joy.

Four days later, the specialist called. I remember exactly. It was almost eight o'clock in the evening, so I wasn't expecting it to be her. She was working late and got a fax. Scott's test results were negative; he was not a carrier. The chances of our kids getting CF were smaller than the chances they would get hit by a bus. That's exactly what she said. It was over. We had been tested for everything possible. I had it all; Scott had none. If I was a cesspool, he was spring water. He said it made him feel better about the whole low sperm count thing. He may have been the problem at first, he said, but he saved us in the end.

For the next two weeks, we laughed at ourselves yet again, laughed at the stupidity of it all, and told anyone who would listen about how genetic counseling was a scam, designed to force unwitting potential parents into expensive, useless testing. We compared ourselves to our next-door neighbors, a lovely couple from Ireland who were also pregnant. They did things differently. She had absolutely no genetic testing, but she did have a glass of wine at least once a week, and in her last week of pregnancy, when the baby wouldn't budge, she downed a pint of Guinness, "to move things along," she said. A week later, she gave birth to an enormous, healthy baby boy with big blue eyes and his father's grin. Her pregnancy was no big deal. We were ridiculous.

Again, I told myself it was time to be happy. As many times as I had tried before to let myself feel the joy of pregnancy, this time it was even harder. I threw myself into work, hoping that by reliving the whole IVF experience through this book, I would somehow get myself back into the pregnancy. Over the next weeks, I slowly let the joy creep back in. I started making lists, lists of things for the babies' room, lists of people to schedule, like the baby nurse and the people from California Closets who would design our changing/dressing room.

By the end of January, work was going well, and I was getting bigger every day. My twenty-four-week checkup went well, and once again my cervix checked out fine. Our next ultrasound was the following Monday, February 4, and my parents were coming down for the weekend to shop for cribs. My mother had never seen an ultrasound, so she was going to stay and go with me Monday to the appointment.

We had a really lovely weekend. We found the perfect cribs and put them on order. We went to a massive baby supercenter and registered for all kinds of fun stuff, like changing pads and diaper genies. The New England Patriots won the Super Bowl, and Scott (a Bostonian) was walking on air. Finally, I felt like the stars were aligned. We were going to have babies. We were going to be parents. I was *really* pregnant. IVF was finally beginning to fade into the past, and parenthood was visible in the future. The nursery would be green with white old-fashioned French country-style cribs. We had even picked our daughter's name.

Monday's ultrasound looked just fine. The babies were growing, the placentas looked good. My mother couldn't tell what she was looking at, but she was beaming anyway. The radiologist told us the babies were each about a pound. That was a great milestone. Then she went to check my cervix with that awful internal probe thing I had come to know and hate. I told her she didn't need to bother, as my ob had checked it digitally the previous Thursday. She told me it was procedure and wouldn't take a minute.

It took more than a minute. As she guided the probe, I could see her bright, cheerful face turn serious. Those few minutes seemed like hours. Before she said a word, I knew we were in trouble.

The technician pulled the probe out and said, "I don't like what I see. I'm going to get the chief radiologist." It seems my cervix had started to shorten. The door was beginning to open, but the babies were nowhere near ready to come out. All my newfound hope suddenly fell away like a drenching rush of water. I felt cold.

That afternoon I rushed back to the ob, who monitored me for contractions but said I had none. She told me to go home and lie down, and we would reassess in a few days. But I'm not the type to wait around well, so I called Dr. Sacks, our fertility specialist. He had gotten us into this, and he was going to get us out of it. Honestly, he was the only one I really trusted with this pregnancy. He referred us to a high-risk neonatologist in Maryland. We saw the specialist the next day. And it was a good thing we did. As he examined me, I had a contraction. We saw it on the monitor. He showed us my son's fist, jammed into my fragile, shortened cervix. We were in trouble.

The specialist said that if I just stayed on strict bed rest, we would have about a 40 percent chance of going to term. If the babies came at twenty-four weeks, they had about a 10 percent chance of survival. Every week I kept them in, he said, would double their chances. Numbers were swimming in my head, and of course none of them made any sense. All I wanted to know was if I was going to lose these precious babies. He obviously could not answer that question.

The specialist recommended surgery, a double "cerclage" to sew up my cervix, plus strict bed rest and a drug called Terbutaline that was thought to help stop contractions, even though there was no real evidence that it did. It was actually an allergy medication, FDA approved for that purpose but not for pregnant women in trouble. I didn't even know that until after I was on it for several weeks. When he suggested it that day, I just said, "Okay, I'll take it." Anything to save those babies.

That Friday I was in the hospital having surgery. It was awful, painful, bloody surgery, but it was done to perfection by the specialist, a man who seemed so calm and so able that I don't even think I asked him where he went to medical school (one of my usual checks on every doctor I see). He was a rock star. He knew it, I knew it, Scott knew it. We never saw him again.

Sunday afternoon I left the hospital, went home to my bed, and shut the door. I shut the door tight. I lay there, flat, with a catheter strung into my thigh delivering large doses of a drug that made my hands shake and my stomach queasy. At first, I thought, maybe I could write. This would be a perfect way to write this book: no distractions. I could be productive, I thought.

But I couldn't do anything but worry. I stared at the ceiling. I watched the game show network. I talked on the phone a little bit, but not much. What did I have to say? What was new? What could I say to anyone who wasn't in my situation, and what could they possibly say to me that I'd want to hear? Every conversation I had may as well have been white noise, so I simply stopped talking.

This was it. This was my punishment for pushing a pregnancy that shouldn't have happened in the first place, I thought. This was what you get for playing God. I talked to Dr. Sacks, and he assured me that the cervix problem had nothing to do with IVF. But in my mind it did. The cervix problem was most likely the result of twins. About 40 percent of women carrying twins have trouble with their cervixes. It's the weight of the pregnancy. Your body miscalculates and starts to contract, thinking that the baby is cooked, when the two are only really half cooked. If I weren't having twins, I probably wouldn't be having this problem. If I hadn't done IVF, I wouldn't be having twins. It all came back to IVF.

I counted every day like it was a year. A cousin of mine, who is a pediatrician, told me that every day in the womb is worth three days in a neonatal intensive care unit. Every day I could keep them in was a victory. I tried to think of it that way. The weeks passed more slowly than any time I can remember. It felt endless. I would not allow myself to think about the babies. I had all the time in the world to read baby books, to order stuff online, to prepare. I did nothing. I canceled California Closets. I didn't want to picture little hanging dresses or little socks in a cubby. A few friends came to visit, but not many. I didn't want to see anybody.

As the contractions continued, and the doctor kept increasing my Terbutaline dose, I felt sicker and sicker. Soon I was forcing my-self to eat—a pregnant woman, forcing herself to eat. This was the ultimate irony. Food is my favorite thing. I've always had something of a weight problem, so I'm careful with food, but I absolutely love to eat. I considered pregnancy to be the food nirvana. Here were nine months during which I was supposed to overeat, supposed to get fat. I'd go on the diet later. I looked forward to the freedom of all those luscious cravings and all those greasy hamburgers that would be "good protein" for my babies. I couldn't even look at a hamburger. Scott tried everything, bringing in French fries, pizza, Cheetos, all my taboo favorites. They all made me ill. Nothing about this pregnancy, *nothing*, was going to be the way I had dreamed of it.

It didn't take long for the anger to set in. I couldn't eat, I couldn't sleep, I couldn't walk around with a big tummy and let people pat it, I couldn't do pregnancy yoga, I couldn't go to Lamaze classes, I couldn't read *What to Expect When You're Expecting* because none of it applied to me. This pregnancy was a fiasco right from the start. Who the hell brings a child into this world by sticking herself full of needles? I had always planned on having this really healthy pregnancy, no caffeine, no alcohol, no sushi. Now I was pumping myself full of some experimental drug that was probably mixing in with all the other things I had shot myself up with at the start and creating some noxious cocktail that would make my babies horribly deformed or sick or just plain stupid. I'm wrong. I wasn't angry. I was enraged.

Now it seems like a strange, surreal blur, as the weeks slowly crept by. I remember little moments, a certain visit from a friend, a trashy novel I lost myself in one day, an obsession with the *$100,000 Pyramid*. I showered once a week for two minutes. I tiptoed to the bathroom when I had to pee and dreaded any time I had to push for a bowel movement. I made sure, as I lay in bed, that my head was never above thirty degrees, as the doctor had ordered. I ate Tums and Zantac like they were candy, as the acid reflux ate away at my throat. Sometimes I cursed my husband. Sometimes I cursed the babies. I mostly cursed myself for being unable to be normal.

Scott did his best. He was actually at his best. He waited on me hand and foot, took care of the house, took care of his work, took care of me and my constant crying fits. He was absolutely positively sure that nothing bad was going to happen to these babies. He decided that the surgeon who had sewn me up at week twenty-four was the greatest surgeon who had ever lived. He had absolute faith. The surgeon had told us the procedure would buy us eight more weeks at the very least, and Scott would neither accept nor even consider anything less. To this day, I don't know how he did it. I've asked him if he was just putting on a good face back then, but I know the answer myself. He believed. He really believed. His optimism was just about the only thing I could count on at the time, and it was probably the only real thing that got me through because I certainly had none of my own.

I remember when I made it to week twenty-eight. That was a milestone because babies have a 90 percent survival rate after week twenty-eight. They survive, but they're very sick. I wanted to go to week thirty-six. With twins, that would be full term enough. Forty weeks is regular full term, but most normal healthy twins don't go that long. Another milestone was week thirty-two. Supposedly they can breathe on their own at week thirty-two, which would be exactly eight weeks after my surgery; if I could just survive this for a few more weeks.

That was the definition of my pregnancy: survival. It was all about waiting, passing the time, surviving the time. My head wasn't filled with visions of round, pink babies swaddled in thick cotton blankets. It was filled with boxes on a calendar: days, weeks, months, all representative of fetal development. Fetal development, not babies. We had this book that gave a day-by-day account of how your baby is developing. I wouldn't let Scott read it every day, only once a week, on the day when we hit a new week of gestation. Somehow it felt like more of an accomplishment that way.

On the fifth day of the thirty-first week the contractions got stronger. The extra Terbutaline hit didn't bring them down, and the nursing service called my doctor, a specialist I had switched to at Georgetown Hospital because I didn't want to have to go all the way to Maryland in an emergency. It was a good thing I switched. The doctor told me to come in immediately.

By the time Scott and I arrived in the delivery area about a half hour later, I was contracting every two minutes. The stitch in my cervix was still holding tight, but the contractions had to be stopped. I was put on a delivery bed and wired up to another drug called Magnesium. This stuff is horrible. It relaxes your muscles so much that you cannot get up at all. The Magnesium slowed the contractions but began to take a toll on my body. I felt like I had a horrible flu.

But the drug was buying me time, enough time to get shots of steroids every twelve hours. These steroids would help the babies' lungs develop more quickly. I made it to Wednesday, and finished the steroids. Wednesday night I started to cough horribly, so much so that I could hardly breathe. The magnesium was relaxing the muscles in my throat so much that it was closing up on me. Thursday morning I went off the Magnesium and back on the Terbutaline. The theory was that the Magnesium had "washed" my system of the Terbutaline, which I had gotten used to, and allowed it to start working again. It worked for about six hours. By Thursday night an overnight resident put me on morphine to stop the pain. By Friday morning the doctor tried Procardia, a blood pressure drug, but the contractions kept coming, and now they were really painful.

The more drugs they put in me, the angrier I got. When was all the drugging going to stop? My mind went back to the IVF. How could these babies survive all the drugs from the beginning and then all these additional drugs at the end? Every time a resident or nurse came in, she would look at the monitors that blipped out my babies' heartbeats and say how great the kids looked. The babies were doing so well! All I wanted to do was shout out: "Hello? There's someone else in this room!" Namely, me.

I had had it. I wasn't afraid anymore. I honestly wasn't. I didn't fear for these babies' lives; I was looking to save my own. I was sick of being stuck with needles and drugs. I was sick of doctors giving me statistics. I was sick of living through a pregnancy that had fought me tooth and nail before it ever even existed. I was sick of trying to feel "normal" when there was nothing normal about all this, when the whole thing was just plain unnatural.

At two o'clock on Friday afternoon, the nurse called my specialist over from his offices. The contractions were getting stronger. He wheeled me in for another sonogram, and the radiologist said, "Something isn't right." In addition to everything, my son's placenta had "abrupted." This is a somewhat rare condition when the placenta starts to come away from the wall of the uterus prematurely. Once again, I had made the cut. The specialist said simply, "How would you like to have your babies today?"

Twenty minutes later I was on the operating table, and at 3:10 and 3:11, Noah Wagner Gold and Madeline Sophie Gold were pulled out via C-section and rushed off to the Neonatal Intensive Care Unit. A large blue sheet had been pulled lengthwise across my chest, so I could see nothing. I heard a tiny cry for a second, and I saw a lot of doctors running around, but that was it. That was the birth. It took forty more minutes for them to sew me back up. After the first five minutes, Scott had been called in to see the babies, so I lay there by myself, a nurse holding my head as I threw up into a plastic bowl.

About two hours later, as my head and stomach spun from all the drugs, I was wheeled in to the NICU to see these two tiny red things, sprawled out under bright white lights. I was afraid to look at them. They were premature by eight weeks, but they were fine, strong, breathing on their own, just over four pounds each.

We won. We beat the odds. My pregnancy was over. We made it—thirty-two weeks and two days.

CHAPTER 13

NORMAL

I had a ridiculous pregnancy. The farther away from it I get in time, the less I even really remember it; somehow it's as if it didn't really exist. No, my pregnancy was not normal, but according to the doctors, once a couple has had success with IVF, medically everything should be normal from then on in, as if the child had been conceived naturally, after some nice Saturday night and a really good bottle of wine.

A study was released in the fall of 2003 (I will discuss more in depth later) about the aftereffects of women who conceive through IVF. Many experience severe depression and difficulty bonding with their IVF children. Although I've not found any studies on the effects of IVF on a still-pregnant mother's emotions, in my own research infertility and IVF played a major role in the actual pregnancy. I think it's like anything you try to do for a long period of time, anything that is deeply emotional and extremely desired. The Oscar winner stands on the stage before the adoring crowd and says over and over, "I can't believe this is happening!" The writer sees a stranger reading his book in a library and the scene is strangely surreal. I've heard of composers who listen to their own music at a concert and suddenly don't recognize a series of bars. I think it's the same. You try so hard for so long and invent the scenario, compose it in your mind. Once it's upon you, it's hard to believe.

Many couples I spoke with felt this way, many did not. For some of the people it was as if IVF were done and gone, and with a quick "Thank you" they never looked back. That's how it was for Tim and Kathy.

> KATHY: I always felt that I was a regular pregnant woman because, just the stages that you're reading about in the books and stuff, I felt good. Every pregnant symptom I was going through, my mother had gone through.
> TIM: She went from talking to her best friend, who had gone through all the science of getting pregnant and IVF and she got all the advice up to that point, and then she swapped over to her mom, who had children naturally, and got the rest of the advice from her. It was like we moved across the street to the next clinic.
> KATHY: You say good-bye, you have your exit visit with the IVF people, and I remember just hugging him. The doctor said, I'll never forget, "Just remember, whatever you have in your mind of how it's going to be, it's going to be better than that."

I was actually surprised at how normal and calm Kathy sounded, unlike yours truly, the constant basket case. She saw IVF as a means to an end and once she got her end the means was no longer important. I envy that more than I could ever explain.

Pregnancy, to make a rash understatement, is an enormously emotional time, and it's not just the hormones either. It's the fact that suddenly you are not just you; you are you and someone else. As obvious as that sounds, it's the most wonderful, horrifying, inexplicable, bizarre feeling that one could ever have. Then, add to it that it took you X number of years, X number of dollars, and X amount of anguish to get there. This experience then can take on, in addition to what I just listed, a distinct fragility unlike anything you've ever experienced. One quarter of normal pregnancies will end in the first trimester, and many of those are in normal, healthy, fertile women. The statistic is not as simple for IVF. For me, yes, it would be the same because our infertility was male factor. But many of the women who are forced to do IVF do it because they had some sort of abnormality in their reproductive system or because they were older. The chances for a successful pregnancy in these scenarios are hard to calculate, but are not the same. All the numbers add up to a pregnancy that, even though a victory, is also, for some, not the end of the game.

ANNE: I spent my first trimester terrified, and then I spent my last trimester terrified, so that was fun too. I was so scared that I was going to lose this pregnancy that I woke up every morning with my heart pounding, looking for blood. So I wasn't really into . . . I couldn't get to babies in the buggy, because that seemed really far away . . . to me.

It was horrible. Pretty much all of it except the only thing I liked, I liked feeling the babies move.

Unfortunately, Anne's fears, like my own, came true.

MICHAEL: It was twenty weeks when they were ready to come out.

ANNE: I had started to dilate. They put in a stitch, cerclage . . . which at that point is surgery. I was on all sorts of drugs throughout my whole pregnancy, fourteen weeks on bed rest.

They went out and ordered the furniture while I was on the bed rest, but I never populated the nursery, in my head. At twenty weeks they told me I would be very lucky to get to twenty-eight weeks. That was going to be the big prize because at twenty-eight weeks you've got a 90 percent survival rate, but the babies are sick. It was horrible.

I had bleeding at eleven weeks. That was a horrible day. I had already started seeing the ob/gyn, but I had just transferred to him, and I called the fertility guy at his office. They came in at 7:00, and I called them at 7:01, and I'm like, "I have to come in," and they said, "Well what do you want us to do for you?"

I said, "I want you to put a sonogram on and I want to see if those hearts are still beating. That's what I want you to do!" And I'm hysterical, and it was 7:15 and I'm in my pajamas driving there. It was horrible.

At one point I'm like, "Okay God, I'd like to miscarry now because I can't spend nine months terrified. I can't do this. I will die. They will die. I'd read all this stuff where the mother's mental attitude impacts the unborn baby, and I'm thinking I'm going to give birth to sociopaths.

Anne didn't lose the babies but at twenty weeks, she had to undergo the same surgery I had to keep them in for as long as possible.

ANNE: By the end of my pregnancy it was me against them. That was a very hideous position to be in. I was so sick, and I knew I had to eat for them. I had terrible reflux. All I wanted to do was sit up, stand up. I was being woken up at night. I felt like I was on fire. I'd never been in so much pain; labor was not that painful. The only thing to do was to stand up. I needed to walk around for an hour, but every step I took I'd be thinking, "I could be killing them, I could be killing them, I could be killing them." I'm thinking, "Do I lie down and I'll die or do I stand up and they'll die?" It was horrible.

I was angry with them, not at IVF, but with them by the time they were born. "You've taken over my body." I'm so sick. I spent my first three months sitting on this couch crying. If we'd adopted, none of that would have happened. Don't get me wrong; I love having natural children. It's great to look at them and see us in them.

Anne had a scheduled C-section at thirty-seven weeks. She was in labor for twelve hours, and after all that bed rest to keep her from dilating, she didn't dilate for all those twelve hours, even on the drug Pitocin. Her children were born healthy and heavy—twin boys.

For Anne, like myself, pregnancy was a battle, not a beautiful time, but in the end it was a victory. People always tell me that they consider me a hero for going through what I did; I still don't understand that because what I did was so totally instinctual. My first experience as a mother, even before the kids were born, was that feeling that I would do anything to protect them. But their birth is a victory and should be seen as such. So many women do what Anne and I did, putting their own health at risk to save their unborn children. I can see that now, but I definitely didn't see it while I was doing it. Alexandra fell somewhere between me and Anne and very practical happy Kathy.

ALEXANDRA: I felt it was so chosen and so sacred and so special. I was like . . . I am a shrine, like I am a museum, this is the most precious pregnancy.

My shaky time was over, I was now a normal person, it was special, but I was not worried about myself. I said to myself, "The worrying is over."

That's not to say I didn't worry at all about miscarriage. I did worry, worried about that in a sense, but I felt like I had been given the greatest gift. I was like this is positive. I felt really positive and I wasn't going to let anything destroy that. I was going through such a thing trying to manage my anxiety with fertility that I was listening to anxiety tapes, and one of the things that I learned was about this concept of . . . I quickly want to finish and tell you that I actually vividly remember Peter over a course of an hour and a half going from the relief into the happy. Like I could see it happen and it was so interesting because I think he got happy before I did. I was still in shock.

I remember we went out to buy food and I was like, I walked down the steps and I was like I am pregnant and I felt so special. I remember him just being like . . . oh, it is such a relief. By the end of the day we were beaming.

Alexandra's pregnancy was relatively easy, despite the fact that she was having twins. She got huge, yes, but she continued working throughout and never had to go on bed rest. Neither she nor Peter ever questioned that IVF had given them anything but normal healthy fetuses.

PETER: I believed in the science. I believed in the placenta and the strength of the uterus; I believed all that.

ALEXANDRA: I knew that I was treated as higher risk because of twins and because of IVF, but I really felt this is going to work for me. This is going to work out, and I remember, when I started with IVF it was all about this concept of "what if" thinking, because all I ever did was "what if" thinking. I walked around, "What if this? What if that?" and so once I was given this gift, I promised myself I was going to step up to the plate and I was going to shake my "what if" thinking and I wasn't going to "what if miscarriage?" and I wasn't going to "what if deformities?" and I was definitely against genetic testing. I said to myself, "Full steam ahead; I am divinely protected." This was my battle and it is over, and I am not going to lose these babies.

KIDS!

CHAPTER 14

NORMAL

I hate the fact that my children are IVF. Sound awful? Tell me about it. It's still true. Yes, I understand the gift I was given. Yes, I feel like a horrible person for even putting that thought in black and white. Yes, I know that if I said that out loud to my husband he would spend the next hour yelling at me and calling me ungrateful. I give it all to you, yes. But I still feel that way.

I hate the fact that in the back of my head I'm always wondering what's around the corner. ICSI is still barely a decade old, which means that the children of ICSI are just reaching puberty. I'm waiting for the studies. I cringe every time I see something about IVF children in the newspaper—and it's not all nuts either. I've already called my fertility specialist twice, after reading articles about how children of IVF are more prone to this type of disease or this type of abnormality. He usually pulls me back from the edge, telling me that this was an inconclusive study or that if my kids did have X, Y, or Z we would have known it when they were born. I still hate it.

I'm not sure if I can blame it on IVF entirely. I had a difficult pregnancy and a difficult birth experience. My children were cut out of my body in an emergency situation, not yet ripe nor ready to come into the world and meet me. I was shivering and dry-heaving when I first heard the tiny cry of my son. When they wheeled me into the Neonatal Intensive Care Unit to see my daughter, I could only look for about a second and a half before I literally screamed for someone to get me the hell out of there. She was this tiny, red, screaming, naked thing, writhing underneath a bright hot light like some inhuman experiment of torture.

I was afraid of my children. They came home on these awful machines called apnea monitors. Heavy, awkward, ancient, VCR-type devices with teeny tiny wires attached to my children's chests with a thick gooey tape that irritated their newborn skin. The machines were monitoring their every breath to make sure that they didn't miss one. Premature babies are prone to apnea. They simply forget to breathe because they're not mature enough to know how to keep doing it. Our children were not put on ventilators, but they did, on occasion, often while eating, stop breathing. To say it was terrifying wouldn't even cover the half of it.

Why is this different than any other early delivery? It's not, but it was the direct result of IVF, and it's very important to understand why. IVF results in an extremely high number of multiple pregnancies and births. According to the CDC, in 2001 29 percent of IVF births were twins and 7 percent were triplets or more. That makes the multiple rate 36 percent for IVF as opposed to 3 percent for normal conception (and this number does not even include traditional non-IVF fertility stimulants). That statistic has serious ramifications that Scott and I knew nothing about when we decided to put two embryos in my uterus. We thought twins would be challenging, but great fun. They certainly are both now, but it's important that every couple embarking on IVF and the inevitable possibility of a multiple pregnancy know the facts.

Half of all twins are born before thirty-seven weeks of gestation (full term is considered forty weeks). In the year 2000, multiple births accounted for 14 percent of infant deaths. Premature birth cannot be taken lightly. According to the March of Dimes, in 2001, the rate of preterm births rose to 11.9 percent, the highest since officials began tracking the category thirty years ago. In the last ten years, the rate of infants born preterm has increased more than 10 percent. No one argues that the culprit is the high number of multiple-fetus pregnancies resulting from IVF. The risks associated with a multiple pregnancy are anemia, urinary tract infection, preeclampsia, postpartum hemorrhage, and cesarean delivery (48.7 percent compared to 17.7 percent for singleton deliveries) to name a few.

Children who are born premature can face a litany of medical problems, from brain damage to cerebral palsy. The average cost of a hospital stay for infants diagnosed as premature starts at $75,000. In 2001, according to the March of Dimes, hospital charges for premature babies totaled nearly $15 billion.

It is because of this dizzying array of numbers and dangers that Great Britain has now taken a legal stand in the IVF debate over multiple births. In March 2004, the Human Fertilisation and Embryology Authority in the United Kingdom, the British body that regulates IVF, ruled that no woman under the age of forty could have more than two eggs or embryos transferred during treatment, regardless of circumstances.

Again, I give all this information not to alarm or frighten, only to educate. I adore being a parent of twins, and my children are a daily gift, but their beginning was difficult, unhealthy, and dangerous. I only wish I had been able to prepare myself for this possibility. Things would have and could have been a lot easier had I simply had more information about premature delivery and premature infants.

In the hospital, each time one of my babies stopped breathing, an unbelievably loud, high-pitched alarm would ring from inside the machine. It could wake the dead, which was, of course, the idea. The doctors kept telling me that it wasn't that big a deal; I was just supposed to wiggle their feet or shake them a bit, and of course they would start breathing again. No big deal. Imagine having to wiggle your children back to life every couple of hours.

My children were in the hospital for the first three weeks of their lives, which is actually a relatively short period of time for children born at thirty-two weeks. Initially the doctors told us they would be there eight weeks, that is, until they reached the forty weeks of a normal gestation. We were very lucky. Our children did remarkably well and suffered no long-term complications. It was because of this that I never regretted what we did. One couple I spoke with, whose IVF twins were also born premature and had far more complications, did turn around and question what they had done. Like me, they didn't really consider the dangers of a twin pregnancy because they were so wrapped up in just *getting* pregnant. Later, the mother had terrible guilt feelings about what her children had to go through physically just to survive those first harrowing months. She felt like it was her fault because she in fact had created the twin pregnancy. Parents of natural twins would never consider this.

I had similar guilt feelings, despite my twins' relative good health, and because of that I pushed myself too hard right from the start. Coming into the hospital every day for three weeks after having a C-section and not being upright for three months was something I can't quite explain because I just don't really remember it. My relatives reminisce about how horrible I looked. I don't know. I don't even know where the weeks went. I don't know what I did when I wasn't in the hospital, but I know I was home a lot because the doctor in the NICU kept telling me to go home and rest. But every time I went home I had this horrible, guilty feeling that I shouldn't be attending to myself; I should be helping my children through their first days, their first breaths, their first movements. I actually thought that if I wasn't there as much as absolutely possible that the nurses in the NICU were going to report me to social services or something, and they would take my children away.

Scott and I had never considered selective reduction, that is, having doctors remove one of the embryos after we knew that they had both become viable. Twins did not seem that abnormal, especially in IVF, and, again, I knew nothing of the risks involved. I was so wrapped up in getting pregnant that the rest was supposed to be easy. I certainly don't regret what I did, and even given their inauspicious beginning, I know I would do it all again, but that doesn't lessen the severity of the experience.

While I was there, visiting my children, I was an emotional basket case. I realize now that a lot of this was because of hormones and fear and fatigue. Still, there I was, failing at breast-feeding, failing at diaper changing, but instead of having all these failures at home, like a normal mother, I was having them in a neonatal intensive care unit, exhausted from the cumulative emotions of infertility, a high-risk pregnancy, and not having stood upright for nine weeks. One time, while feeding my tiny daughter, she spit up what seemed to me like an enormous amount of milk, and then her alarm began to shriek. The nurse just stood there, expecting me to follow the procedure she had taught me and shake her little feet, which I was doing. But I had no idea she was already breathing again. I started to scream. I actually shouted out, "Help!" I think that's the only time I've ever done that for real. I will never ever forget that feeling. If not the panic, the feeling continued through much of the first few months of my children's lives.

I remember one of the interviews I did with an IVF couple, the same one in which the mother expressed terrible guilt about her premature twins. I considered it the least fruitful and decided not to use it. All my questions about IVF seemed rather irrelevant to these parents. I followed my outline of issues, but for each one I got little to no useful insights. The couple kept saying they couldn't remember or they just didn't know how they felt. All they remembered was dealing with premature twins. It was horribly frustrating.

But later, after my kids were born, I remembered a phrase the couple kept using: "Well, that wasn't such a big deal, compared to the whole preemie issue." I had never really focused on that, probably because I did the interview before my children were born. Now I get it. I totally get it. IVF is nothing compared to dealing with premature babies, but dealing with premature babies that are the result of IVF creates a whole new set of emotions, guilt being the leader.

Living through the first year of a premature child's life is a never-ending flow of fear, uncertainty, vulnerability, and heartache. Your child barely responds to you for the first few months; she doesn't even start acting like a newborn until she has reached the time she was actually supposed to be born. Newborns aren't exactly the most responsive creatures. Any parent knows you really don't get much back for those first months. Imagine extending that time period indefinitely. You're never sure exactly when to start treating your child as normal and, consequently, you don't for quite a while.

To me, the very fact that my children were preemies was due to the very fact that they were IVF. The logic was simple. If I hadn't done IVF, then I wouldn't have been pregnant with twins, and if I weren't pregnant with twins, I never would have had the problems I did with my pregnancy, and my children wouldn't have been born two months early.

My husband, Scott, felt none of this. Yes, he had the same concerns about the children being so tiny and so weak at first, but his always-optimistic side kicked in immediately, and he saw all their accomplishments, while I saw all their failings. He would always remind me to use their "corrected age," that is, the age they were chronologically minus the eight weeks they were premature. By that calculation, he would say, they were doing everything right on track. While I used to dread coming into their room in the morning and starting a day of tense feedings and endless crying, he described it as "Christmas morning!" nearly every day. I admire this ability in him, but I could never find it within myself.

Adding to the stress of it all, my daughter had reflux. She spit up what seemed to me like most of what I gave her, and the burning sensation in her throat made her cry nearly every moment she was awake. The doctors gave her drugs, which I couldn't stand. I know that her reflux had nothing to do with IVF. My older brother had terrible reflux forty-two years ago, my mother reminded me. It's not even necessarily a result of prematurity, but it exacerbated an already difficult situation and chipped away hourly at any sense of control I was trying to achieve. Plus, I just didn't want her on any more drugs.

Before my kids were even conceived, there were drugs. Once they were conceived, and my pregnancy went bad, there were more drugs. Now they were born and I was supposed to be giving my tiny little girl even more serums with more names I couldn't pronounce. I couldn't do it. I'd take her off them, then put her back on, then get a new drug. It was ridiculous. Her brother was gaining weight rapidly, while she was spitting up everywhere and gaining weight much slower.

Interestingly, I found that some of the couples I interviewed had quite the opposite view of IVF's relationship to "normal." They thought IVF made their kids better, stronger, faster.

> ALEXANDRA. My feeling is like they are bionic, because they were made in a lab and they survived those conditions, and they rose to the top, ahead of their class, and they were such good, strong embryos.
> PETER: I had general father fears, I am sure, but after the first sonogram, they said no cleft lip, two arms, two legs on each baby. I would've had those fears no matter what, because you can have that no matter how they are made. I am a believer in science. You've got a great track record. And these are $5,000 babies!

Tim and Kathy felt the same way, but Kathy admitted to me that when her son had a kidney problem, she thought first of the IVF. Did it have something to do with the illness? Her doctor assured her no, but, like me, her first intuition was to question the IVF.

> TIM: The only thing that ever crossed my mind was when they chose which embryos to implant. He took the best

ones, so he was playing with nature in that sense, where he chose the strongest-looking ones, and that's different than if one of the others had made it in naturally.

KATHY: It's not about IVF anymore. I haven't even thought of it . . . until you brought the project to us. We're so busy with the baby now . . . trying to get down a routine, trying to get used to being a mom.

Anne and Michael considered their twin boys nothing short of extraordinary.

MICHAEL: My mind goes to the other side of the discussion, which is, okay, these guys are going to come out stronger because they've gone through this rugged process. I said, "Well, they will come out different and stronger in some ways and maybe not so strong in others," but I tend not to spend a lot of time on questions that really don't have much of an answer, and even if you did get the answer, what then?

But what about questions that do have an answer, questions about who your children really are. Without genetic testing, no father can ever be 100 percent sure that their child is truly their own. Every mother can, every mother except an IVF mother. Identity becomes inflated when you're battling infertility. Any couple who goes through infertility inevitably considers adoption at some point, and the whole issue of identity is center stage. Will I be able to love a child that isn't genetically mine? I strongly believe that because infertile couples have already gone the identity route, it plays a much larger role in the IVF process.

IVF, as I've already said, is an out-of-body experience. You have to have an enormous amount of trust and faith in people whom you barely know and people you will never meet. Your doctor takes your most valuable possession, your eggs and your sperm, and gives them to a technician whose job it is to create an embryo, to make a life.

Who are these people? Why do they do it? Is it totally routine to them? These are questions you don't always ask because you're too busy asking, "Will it work? Will it work?" It's only afterward, when you look into the eyes of your newborn babies and search for that piece of yourself that you've waited so long to see, that you suddenly wonder, did they do it right? Most of the couples I spoke with said this possibility had at least crossed their minds.

And it's not irrational. In 1995, a doctor at the University of California, Ricardo Asch, was accused of taking his patients' fertilized eggs and putting them in other women's uteruses. He was considered one of the top in his field, but after he was indicted, he ran away to Mexico. In 1992, Cecil Thompson, MD, a doctor in Virginia, was convicted of "anonymous donor" fertilization. He used his own sperm in at least seventy-five cases. These are hideous criminal instances of fraud, to say nothing of the possibility of innocent mistakes in the laboratory. I thought about this a lot, and I know I'm not alone.

Scott thinks I'm ridiculous. He says he has no question at all in his mind that our twins are our twins and no one else's. My daughter looks exactly like me; everyone says it. She actually looks a lot like my father. But my son is harder to place. Scott swears Noah looks like him, and some other people have commented that way, but I don't see it. My son is beautiful, strong, even tall for his age (and Scott is six foot four), but I often find myself searching for a sign. So far, all I can see is that he has inherited my love of music.

So why don't I just have them tested and be done with it? I can't decide which reason carries more weight: that I'd feel too ashamed, or that I'm afraid I'd realize my worst nightmare. What if they weren't mine? Could someone take them away? What if they were half mine and half someone else's? I don't think I could deal with the consequences, so I won't have them tested. But, again, my relationship with them is not as easy as it could be.

I've already said that bonding with my children did not come easily for me. I've blamed it on the way they were born, the fact that they were born early, but this one really wins out. Because of the way they were conceived, I feel less connected to them somehow. They were not conceived inside of me, like most kids. It even goes beyond my fear of a mistake in the laboratory; it's more like someone gave me these things, put them inside me, and then told me to believe that they were my children. A doctor did that, whereas for most normal people, God does that.

In some ways, I feel as if it's even harder than adoption. When you adopt a child, you know he's not genetically yours, and you accept that from the start and move on. With IVF, you have to believe. You have to trust. And if you're a skeptical, untrusting nut like myself, that can eat away at the most natural of relationships and cause a type of guilt that is really too hard to explain. I love my children. I would do anything for them. I think about them all day, I worry, I wonder, I dream of their futures; most of it is normal. But then there's that nagging part that isn't.

Every couple I spoke with who had children through IVF said yes, of course, they had considered the possibility of a mistake in the laboratory.

KATHY: We always joked, oh, honey, who's he going to look like, probably the UPS man! They probably mixed up the embryos. You always say stuff like that, like he's going to come out black. We joke about that because he could. There could be a mix-up in the lab. That's a way of life, even though they have their procedures in place.

Anne and Michael joked as well, but the reason it didn't bother them so much was because they didn't consider parenting and bonding necessarily a genetic right.

ANNE: We used to joke that the babies would come out looking like our doctor. But these babies are clearly ours. Trevor looks exactly like he does in his baby pictures and Alex looks exactly like I do in my baby pictures. We feel pretty confident that they're ours.

One of the reasons I was so into adopting is, I've always been 100 percent convinced that how you got the baby didn't matter and that once you had the baby it was yours. I didn't bond with my children or love my children because I carried them, and I didn't fall in love with them because they carry my genetic code. You fall in love with them because you have a daily relationship with them.

I do believe nature over nurture in terms of how they end up turning out, but in terms of how I feel about them,

I actually think I would have bonded a lot faster with non-natural children.

Alexandra thought about doing genetic testing. She and Peter tell a funny story about the day Alexandra's eggs were fertilized:

PETER: We collected my sample at home, but I could've collected it . . .

ALEXANDRA: In the parking lot.

PETER: The sample was in a bag on the floorboard of the car at 5:30 in the morning, a January morning, as we drove up to Rockville, Maryland. Well it should have been under someone's arm or something like that apparently. We got there, and some ratty looking . . . nurse says, "Okay we need a sample from you, and I said, "Oh, no, we've got it right here," and she says, "Oh well, put that under your arm," or something. So right there was that anxiety that they're not going to be good anymore. Then they take the sample. Our doctor takes Alexandra away and sucks the eggs out, and I am in the waiting room while that is happening, and the lab technician comes out in a coat and says, "Are you Mr. Roberson? We need you to give us a sample." I said I gave one. I gave the nurse one two hours ago, and sat there and fretted and then the doctor came out about fifteen minutes later and said Alexandra was fine, he took twenty-one eggs out. I said someone just asked me if I had a sample. I brought it in early this morning, could you make sure they got it and they know where it is. He disappears in the back and came out and he's like everything is okay. But you can imagine, I mean, I believe everything is okay, but come on, how goofy can you get?

What were all the jokes about our doctor's baby?

Despite all their joking, Alexandra did consider DNA testing on her twins.

ALEXANDRA: I was. I literally was, and then I lost my nerve. I felt like everyone would think like that was, I would darken the party.

Both Alexandra and Peter were so impressed by the IVF process and by the science that fears of mistakes soon abated.

ALEXANDRA: It was the coolest process. I said to Peter, even if this doesn't work out, just that we had to witness this process. It is so cool and it is just a real slice of life, you know, I thought this is really amazing, and I said to Peter, thousands of dollars later, for all we know, they just put coffee grounds in me. We're both like, what do you know?

But once they saw their twins, they knew. They could see themselves in their children, and, more important, they could see the gift that was given them. They didn't want to question anymore; they just wanted to enjoy. They were finally ready to be normal. I envy that.

CHAPTER 15

AFTEREFFECTS

For some people, IVF ends at conception. For others, a little more apprehensive, it ends with birth. And for others still, it never ends. It's not necessarily the lack of normalcy that I've already addressed, but the results of a different way of starting babyhood as well as the physical and emotional aftereffects of the process.

There are several aftereffects of IVF, number one being what to do next if the IVF is unsuccessful. Then, for those who are successful, there is the challenge of raising twins, triplets, quads. There are also issues to be considered down the road, like what do you do with extra embryos, and do you tell your children how they were conceived? Many of these are issues that you don't think about when you are in the throes of a fertility battle. How can you? Fighting for fertility is such an all-engrossing, all-consuming situation, that it often leaves little time or energy for thought about what follows.

To be honest, I never considered adoption, probably because we were successful with IVF on the first try. Unlike some others I spoke with, I always assumed I'd be able to have children naturally, so I didn't think about adoption any time before I was married. Even when our troubles began, I don't think I wanted to think about adoption. Since Scott had sperm, and I had eggs, I always figured we could make it work. I know I've said that I had a hard time believing that I actually finally did get pregnant, but I also had an even harder time considering adoption. Not so for Carol and Mike and Chris and Kate. They didn't have a choice.

After a decade of hope and heartache, Carol and Mike had to call it quits. They had been through groundbreaking procedures in medicine, successfully extracted epididymal sperm from Mike, and spent thousands and thousands of dollars. Carol's body simply rejected every embryo that was implanted. They were tapped out, financially and emotionally. The roller-coaster was over. They were getting off.

MIKE: I was probably a little stronger on it than Carol was, but it was pretty much a joint decision.

CAROL: Well, you come to the realization that if you want a child there are only X number of ways you're going to get some. If you can't have them, the only option is to adopt them, unless you kidnap them, and I wasn't about to go there.

Immediately we said we were going to do foreign adoption, we're not messing around here. That had always been part of the fear with all the cases where one biological parent comes back.

MIKE: There had just been a big case out in the Midwest where the biological father came back and wanted the kid and said he never signed releases and all that.

CAROL: That would just be the absolute last straw.

MIKE: And we knew with all the luck that we'd been having that it would probably happen to us.

They weren't taking any chances, so they went to an agency that specialized in Russian adoptions. They didn't speak the language. They didn't know much about the country or its culture, but in that foreign land they found their family and finally put IVF behind them.

MIKE: I won't say that it wasn't worth it to give IVF the shot, but I will tell you, and I am not a good Presbyterian, and I don't believe in predestination, but the day that we sat in the orphanage in Novosibirsk, and they brought those kids in and plopped them down on our laps, it was right. I just knew that that was supposed to be.
CAROL: From the day we came home with them, everybody just said, "Your daughter looks like you! This is unreal!"

I love these kids dearly, but I guess if we'd had an option to have our own, that would have been the number one choice, but we tried, and it didn't work.

Chris and Kate first thought about using a surrogate. Kate's sister was ready and willing, but that was a huge leap to take.

KATE: I asked my sister, and she had mentioned it. So Chris and I talked about it and we decided that if we were to use her eggs, that would be kind of weird; it would be Chris's and my sister's baby, but I asked her and she went to her doctor, and her doctor said, "Your sister's young, she really shouldn't be giving up yet, and it might not be the best thing for you." Of course my sister just went on to have her fifth child at age thirty-eight, so obviously she could have done it. But that would have been a lot to ask of my sister because being pregnant is scary, and things can go wrong.

CHRIS: The desire was for us to have a child that was both Kate's and mine.

KATE: He didn't want it to be just half him and half somebody else.

CHRIS: This was our thing, and if it wasn't going to be Kate and me, then it wasn't the package I was looking for.

Choosing a surrogate or donor eggs, I've found, is an impossibly personal choice. There are some, like Chris and Kate, who couldn't picture it. And then there are others who can and do. I know of more than one couple who used donor eggs or donor sperm or surrogates. A woman stopped me on the street shortly after my twins were born and asked all about the brand of double stroller I was using. She was a small, slim fortysomething woman, and she easily announced that her twins were arriving in six weeks. Obviously, she wasn't pregnant. She and her husband had used a surrogate. I don't know if the eggs or the sperm or both were theirs, but this woman could not have been more excited about preparing for motherhood. Later, when I'd see her and her kids and her husband in the park, they seemed like a normal happy family, dealing with all the trials and tribulation of raising twins. No difference.

When using donors, it is obviously hardest on the person who is left out of the equation, but from what I've heard at least, once the baby is born, the love becomes unconditional. Parenthood seems more instinctual than genetic. In more than one instance, I've seen couples go on to have additional children with the help of donors and surrogates. Still, it's not for some, and it wasn't for Chris and Kate.

CHRIS: At that point I was starting to get kind of bitter. I was obsessing, constantly trying to refigure how much money did . . . we put into the whole thing.

KATE: I mean it was like twenty grand.

CHRIS: It was more than that because you've got the mini-IVF for nine thousand but then you have five thousand more in the drugs on top of that. And that's when I said okay, because there are also a lot of hidden costs, not so much hidden but costs, just even when you look at the co-pay, you know when you go to the doctor so often.

KATE: And you know it's $25 every time you go to the doctor and you're seeing the doctor an awful lot. We spent twenty grand to try to get pregnant.

We would not have been able to do IVF again and then adopt. I mean at that point we're thinking, we could refinance the house and we can come up with thirty grand. It's not like we could come up with thirty and then three, six, nine months later come up with another thirty. You can only refinance your house so much; you can only get so much equity out of it.

CHRIS: And also at that point in time, even though we didn't have the money, that wasn't driving our decision.

KATE: It was about us being parents, it was about us having a child, and it was no longer about us having a biological child. We wanted a child and we wanted to be parents and it didn't matter anymore if it was ours.

CHRIS: We knew we'd be good parents.

KATE: Right, and so at that point we said, you know what, there's a baby out there already and why not go give that child a home and a good life because ultimately that's what we want. We want a baby, we want to be parents, and it just doesn't matter if that baby is biologically our child.

CHRIS: Once you get over that idea that you're not going to have a child, or you're going to have to go through an awful lot more before you have a child that is from you, once you got beyond that, which didn't take that much for Kate and I, so it must have been there all along.

KATE: It was for me all along.

Chris and Kate finally got their child, and Carol and Mike got two at the same time! Imagine adopting, and then imagine adopting two? The first months of parenthood are tough for anyone, but I think for anyone with twins, it is harder. I absolutely love the fact that I have twins. But Scott and I have a saying: twins aren't twice as hard as one child, they're about three times as hard! Why? Because it's not just two babies, it's two babies plus this entity that is the twin relationship. It's trying to give each child as much personal attention as you can while always feeling guilty that you're neglecting the other. It's trying to teach sharing and waiting when you've never even tried teaching yes and no. If the average new parent feels like an idiot, the average twin parent feels like an idiot's charity case.

As hard as it is to be the parents of twins under any circumstances, IVF parents of twins can have additional and unique emotional problems. In the fall of 2003, at the annual meeting of the American Society for Reproductive Medicine, a team of Harvard University researchers presented a fascinating study of the parents of IVF twins, "Multiple Birth Family Outcomes," published by Harvard Medical School. The purpose of the study was to determine if multiple births resulting from IVF "impact maternal well-being and family quality of life."

According to the study:

Even with the high socioeconomic status of this sample, multiple births resulted in significant increases in unmet family needs, social stigma, and higher maternal depression scores. In addition, multiple births resulted in significant decreases in maternal quality of life and health and functioning, satisfaction with their marriage and their husband and lower overall quality of life scores. Multiple births also resulted in more negative appraisals of their decision to seek treatment, and of reproductive science. Finally, multiple births resulted in a trend towards significantly more negative evaluations of their treatment outcome.

This study was published well after the birth of my own twins, and when I first read it I did so with not a little bit of validation. I experienced many of the same symptoms described above, but I didn't know that they could have something to do with IVF. I thought I was just failing at being a good mother. Failure, in fact, was the overriding emotion throughout my children's first year. I realize that plenty of new parents feel this way regardless of their circumstances, but I always felt that my situation was more severe than others. Again, the first year is hard for any parent, but I was so completely unhappy, so unable to experience joy. Anne had a similar experience.

ANNE: We came home on New Year's Eve. That was the worst night of my life. The night we took them home. We had no idea. Feeding was this long, drawn out . . . I never really did get the hang of doing them both at the same time. They were not great nursers.

MICHAEL: Was I angry at the fact that we ended up with twins? I think through a combination of when you're dealing with sleep deprivation, you might think some thoughts that you might not otherwise think logical in a sane world. But the connection never goes multilayer. I could be angry, angry at lack of sleep, angry at a lot of things, mostly angry at nothing, just angry, but never take it to the next level of angry at the children. No, angry at the process that brought the children to the world. For me it was too far removed.

ANNE: I had severe postpartum depression. I had a lot of problems. I'm fairly convinced that it ruined my health. I spent three years on fertility drugs. I'm convinced that . . . the only place IVF came up was, I was told that, I never did make enough milk for two, and I was told, again anecdotally, that IVF mothers of twins seem to have that problem a lot, whereas natural mothers of twins don't. That's what the lactation consultant told me. Again, anecdotal, no proof, no scientific study.

I'm also convinced that three years of pumping myself full of fertility drugs had a lot to do with my depression.

MICHAEL: We had a great marriage, and the most trouble we've ever had were in the first twenty-four months of parenthood, without question, and it was for a variety of reasons: her health being part of it, broadly speaking, but just the stress and strain of two very intense kids.

If I can speak absent the knowledge of the health ramifications on my wife, then I would say I would definitely go through it again. They're worth it. I will also say that there have been plenty of times when we've said, "We had a really good life, just the two of us."

ANNE: There were times in the first year, for sure, if you'd asked us, would you have wanted to have kids . . . When I was pregnant, I was so fat, dumb and happy. Everybody's like, "It's going to be so hard," and I said, "We don't have any other kids. We won't know anything else." It's not so hard to figure out when you're up in the middle of the night with two screaming babies that if you only had one it would be a lot easier.

Anne and I had similar experiences, and perhaps that's because we also had similar pregnancies. I constantly marvel at the people who seem so ready for twins and so unflappable once they arrive. I've not found any studies that link fertility drugs to lactation problems, but there is new evidence coming out every day that there may be some other aftereffects. Because the studies are new and some ongoing, I would rather leave these findings to the science journals, but suffice it to say there are concerns. The drug protocols today are not what they were in the beginning, and because so many people are now doing IVF two, three, and four times, the cumulative effects of these drugs can be dangerous. Some studies are linking them to cancer and irreversible bone loss. Again, much of this is uncharted territory, and for many many people there are absolutely no negative side effects.

Alexandra was like that. She and Peter saw their twins as the greatest gifts they could ever receive, and Alexandra was armed with research, insight, and schedules. She had her kids trained to eat, sleep, and poop exactly when she wanted them to—by ten weeks old! She was the most together new mother I'd ever seen and she made it look so simple; she actually breast-fed her twins for more than six months! I barely made it ten weeks, and that was just pumping, because I totally failed at actual breast-feeding.

Still, despite all that sense of control, Alexandra and Peter weren't prepared for one aftereffect of IVF: fertility. You've heard the story before, and you will hear it again and again. I spoke with Alexandra shortly after her twins' first birthday. I wanted to see how all the festivities went and get some tips on planning my own first party. I knew the moment I heard her voice that something was off. She didn't sound her usual together self. She sounded like she was about to fall apart.

Before I could even ask what was up, Alexandra blurted out, "Please don't tell anybody, because we're not three months yet, but you're not going to believe this: I'm pregnant."

Frankly, I was more shocked that she was actually having sex. I have to admit, Scott and I may as well have been comatose roommates the first year of our twins' lives. But yes, Alexandra and Peter, through no work of a doctor, through no drugs, through no intention, were eight months away from baby number three. That July, after what Alexandra described as a more uncomfortable, nauseating pregnancy than her first, she and Peter welcomed a little girl to their already busy home. I saw them about three months into their new adventure, and Alexandra looked thin and harried.

"I'm like a refugee," she said. "I'm running around, trying to survive, and I'm just begging somebody to feed me."

I gave her a bagel. What else could I do?

I don't know if there's some scientific reason, or maybe it's a stress thing, or maybe it's just God's little comedy routine, but I know of more than one, actually more than five couples who went through years of infertility, did IVF successfully, and then shortly thereafter were surprised by a natural pregnancy.

Some doctors will tell you that it's easier to conceive a second child, especially soon after the birth of the first, because the woman's body is still surging with all kinds of happy maternal hormones. But I also wonder if, given this prevalence, perhaps many of us don't jump into IVF too quickly. Our specialist did tell me and Scott that we did have a chance of getting pregnant naturally. He said it could take five years or less or more, but it could definitely happen. IVF didn't exist when Scott's parents were trying, so they just kept trying, for about five years, and eventually he was conceived. Interestingly, his sister was conceived barely two years after that.

The popularity of IVF is also due to the fact that so many women today are trying to get pregnant later in life. I was already thirty-four when we started considering IVF. The thought of waiting five years, when my natural fertility would be diminishing anyway, didn't seem like an option. Or perhaps it's the instant gratification of our current society that makes waiting no longer as plausible. If you can order just about anything in the world you could possibly want online and then, through expedited delivery, get it the next day, how are you supposed to wait an indeterminate number of years for something as important as a child?

The question is: Is it wrong? Has IVF become so run-of-the-mill that it's barely a consideration before we jump right in? Well, on the one hand, if you've got the money, then why not? But on the other hand, as usual, I have to go back to my basic fears that an IVF child might not be as healthy and normal as a natural child. If that's so, then are we rushing parenthood to the detriment of our own children? I'm guessing most fertility specialists would say absolutely not, but I still wonder. I really don't even remember considering IVF and its ramifications so much before we did it. We had done three IUIs and our specialist said that if we really wanted a child right away, we should be more aggressive. It just seemed like the next step. Infertility was so difficult and so emotionally suffocating that I think both Scott and I just wanted to take every breath we could, and IVF was a big gulp. Maybe it was just something different than what we were already doing, which clearly wasn't working. I wish now that I had thought about it more. I'm sure we would have done IVF regardless, but I really never prepared myself emotionally for what was to come.

Our specialist's office did recommend a counselor, but I thought that was for couples who were having marital problems related to infertility. It never crossed my mind that this person was there to help us with the whole package, all we were about to get ourselves into. How could I have known? I never realized that IVF was more than a medical procedure. I often wonder now why that never occurred to me.

I recently had lunch with a colleague who doesn't know how my children were conceived. He's not married, nor does he have children. Somehow we got onto the topic of cloning, and in passing, he said he didn't believe in all the new fertility procedures either. He suggested that if a couple was unable to have children it was simply life's or God's or whatever's way of saying that they shouldn't reproduce. He said adoption should be the only recourse to infertility. I didn't say anything to him about my twins, but I admit I took it very hard. My first instinct was to hate him instantly, but anger turned again to my own insecurities. I don't believe he is right. I actually think him quite ignorant and reckless in his opinions, but he released a few demons in me that I thought I'd finally buried. Those are the demons that whisper: "Who are you to play God?"

He went on to say that it appalled him to think of how many frozen embryos there are sitting in Sub-Zeros all over the country. This has actually become quite the popular issue to discuss, often in the context of cloning or designer babies. I saw a piece on *The Today Show* recently about this. The story was about egg donations to infertile couples and the custody issues that could arise.

In asking my couples about what they would do with their leftover embryos, I found the answers as varied as the couples. There are really four options with embryos: use them again yourself, destroy them, donate them to science for stem cell research or the like, or donate or sell them to an infertile couple. Tim and Kathy, both Catholic, said they could never destroy their ten remaining embryos; they see them as potential life and, therefore, life.

> TIM: The simple answer is that we're going to have them implanted. That's probably the most agreeable solution. That to me is the most respectful thing and probably the simplest answer for anybody who would have issues with what to do with them.

KATHY: A lot of people say, "Go fresh, not frozen" but we want to try with those other ones because when I was pregnant, riding around in the car, and I'd pass the building where they're stored, I'd go, "That's where my family is, that's where all his brothers and sisters are!"

TIM: Driving by that place, I tell people, "That's the most expensive singles bar in Rhode Island!"

KATHY: You always think that they're in there, you know, and I don't really have hassles about it or a head case about it. I just know that we're definitely going to try to use them, definitely.

A friend of ours always said, "Destroy them." But we would rather give them to somebody else, if we didn't use them ourselves, because we know how happy it made us, and the fact that they might have our physical characteristics, I'm okay with that because I know how much an IVF baby is wanted. I think we'd give them to somebody else before we'd give them to science.

TIM: I don't know about giving them to science, even though I know how important that is. This is where real issues come into play.

KATHY: Real issues come into play after you've had the baby and realize okay, look, I've got nine embryos or ten embryos sitting in a vault and what do I do with the other ones?

It's definitely weird to give them away, but what about people who have no eggs? We're not there yet so we don't really know.

TIM: We've benefited from this greatly, and we respect it and it is a special, special gift that we've been given. In a way, to stand up and say, "I'd offer this to someone else" is probably one of the best things I could do. Yes, it could be different or strange that there would possibly be one of our children running around out there with other parents and has a whole separate life than ours. That is kind of an odd thing to accept, but you know that the parents would really want to have that baby and would probably go to any measure. If they did take one of our embryos, that would be a last-ditch effort for them, because they'd probably tried everything else. So you know these would not be just some random folks, so that makes it a little easier.

KATHY: I think to destroy is worse than to donate. Some people don't feel comfortable with it, so destroying is the only option for them.

TIM: Having them destroyed is not the option, and I think we agree on that, that won't happen. I'm just a little queasy about the science thing, even though I know what the uses are there. I'd rather see them used for babies.

I'm not sure Scott and I are as generous. We often joke about our nine embryos on ice, our little baseball team in the freezer. We have both agreed that we can't give them to another couple. The idea of our children running around out there without us ever knowing them is just not an option for either of us. It's ironic, given all my fears about mix-ups in the lab, that I would feel this way about microscopic organisms, but go figure, I do. I don't think we would use them either. For one thing, my pregnancy was so bad that my doctor has told me it would be very dicey for me to carry another child, not to mention twins.

Science is usually the route Scott and I favor most when we talk about it (we have been remarkably slow to come to any firm decision). Of course, cynical me is still concerned that something would go awry in the donation, and the embryos would actually end up being donated to some couple, and my kids would end up living their lives without me.

Stem cell research, I believe, is the most noble option. There are already so many living people out there who could benefit from the science that isn't it worth donating the potential of life to these already existing lives? Given that we would probably destroy the embryos rather than use them, science seems the best option. Of course, I wonder what a child of IVF might think of that? What would my children think if I were to tell them that they had nine brothers and sisters, but I chose not to bring them into this world?

Besides that, what would any IVF child think of how they themselves were brought into this world? This is yet another aftereffect that some parents will choose to confront and others will never reveal. What do we say when our children inevitably ask, "Where did I come from?"

ANNE: First of all, I want them to know how wanted they were. We worked hard to get them. These weren't love children conceived in the back of a car. We very much wanted children.

MICHAEL: Plus she's Jewish, there's that guilt thing she's got working in there somewhere.

ANNE: I don't think I will tell them how miserable I was. I won't tell them that part, but I will tell them that we went to lengths. The reason I would do that is because I have a friend who seems to derive a great deal of joy from the fact that her parents, thirty-five years ago, went through some fertility things to get pregnant with her. She gets all puffed up and says, "They really wanted me!" If I could give that to my kids, great!

ALEXANDRA: I will tell them because it is reality and because it is a miracle and we want them to know that they are a miracle.

PETER: Besides, we have that photo, and I have always wanted to have the embryo photo, sonogram photo, and baby photo.

ALEXANDRA: My feeling is that they should know that we fought for them.

PETER: And maybe they'll be a little more grateful.

ALEXANDRA: And they'll know that it is a perfectly good way to come into the world and I am not ashamed and we proselytize IVF in the street because we want people to be saved from infertility if they can be and we, in a way, it was the best thing that ever happened to us.

Once we found out we were pregnant we told everybody. Everyone is like oh twins! And then say . . .

PETER: I say they were engineered.

ALEXANDRA: And I say yes, we had a long fertility battle, we felt lost, we get to have twins and it's so great and I have always wanted twins. I told everyone right away.

KATHY: When we tell him down the road how he got here, we're going to just tell him how much he was wanted and loved and how we all waited for him and had to wait and wait and wait. It was extra special, definitely.

TIM: We just had to go to extreme measures to get him. We wanted him so bad. It's kind of like a person who can't see and has to put on glasses.

I feel the same way. I imagine it might be a bit strange for a person to know that she was conceived in a laboratory, but it's not as if she would remember it or remember her birth or childhood any differently than any other child. And isn't it a greater gift for a person to know how very much she was wanted?

We all spend our lives searching for love, wanting to be needed. As cold and scientific as IVF is, the force of desire behind it embodies all the love and need a continent full of children could ever wish for. To persevere through infertility, to seek out every road possible, to endure the waiting, the pain, the disappointment, and the uncertainty is proof of a love and a hope that no child could ever question. Yes, I will tell my children how they were conceived. I will tell them how much their father and I wanted them. They will know that we needed them as much as they needed us.

CHAPTER 16

LOOKING BACK

How can you look at a beautiful, loving, bright-eyed child and ever say that you regret how he came into this world? How can you say that the creation of a life isn't worth every penny, tear, and cry of pain expended? I think of all the people in this world who had difficult childbirths or who gave birth to children with illnesses or even children who died. Would they ever say they regret having had those children? Probably not.

When I asked most of my couples if they regretted doing IVF, most answered with a resounding no. Most looked at me like I was crazy even to ask. But there were some, there were some who paused, some who looked a little guilty for a moment, and some who had the courage to say yes out loud. Anne was one of those people.

ANNE: Despite the fact that two years later, this couldn't be more of a success story. And our kids, by the way, are fabulous. People stop us in the street constantly. They're just really special kids. Having said all that, if I knew then what I know now, I'm almost sure I wouldn't have done it, that I would have adopted from the beginning. I would never have gone through the process.

If somebody had come to me in the beginning and said, "IUIs aren't going to work for you. If you want to do this, you need to do IVF," it's a toss-up as to whether or not I could've emotionally done it, just from the fear factor.

Three years? That's a long time. I did many, many IUI cycles. I don't know if I would've been open to IVF then because I was afraid of it, and I needed those three years to get used to the idea. I probably just would have said, "I'm not doing that, let's adopt." I would have children. I don't know that I'm ever going to be . . . I have to take drugs today that I didn't have to take before I do all this to feel an approximation of how I used to feel.

Anne's husband, Michael, was not as quick to say he wouldn't have done it, but he, of course, wasn't the one shooting himself up with drugs, and now he wasn't the one trying to survive the aftereffects of all those drugs. He said that except for the health effects on Anne, he had no regrets.

I found it extremely courageous of Anne to be able to tell me that. She obviously adores her twin sons. Their house is a testament to that; every corner of their world says kids, from the gorgeous mural she had painted on the wall of their nursery, to the dining room crammed with three different models of strollers to the toys, toys, toys everywhere. But it's important to know, and Anne recognizes that IVF isn't for everyone. While I haven't seen any medical studies, Anne is living proof that the drugs can have aftereffects. Perhaps it's not even the drugs, but the stress and strain of going through a medical process for years that leaves a person drained, depressed, even angry. I believe it can happen, and I thank Anne for giving fair warning.

I expected to hear regret from the couples who did not succeed at IVF, but Carol and Mike surprised me. Imagine trying something for ten years and still believing it was the right thing to do! Their only regret is that science was not as advanced when they tried it, and they often wonder if they would have been successful, had they tried IVF today.

MIKE: I don't fault science.

CAROL: I don't either.

Who knows, now there's this new procedure, they let the embryos go to eight cells. Maybe if there had been eight cells maybe they would have implanted. There's always this maybe, maybe the next step would have been the right one. Well, we didn't have the option. It was just a big depressing mess for a long time.

MIKE: We didn't have much of a marriage for ten years.

CAROL: We can answer people's questions on both sides of going through it, and I know that protocols have changed, some parts aren't as bad as we encountered when we were doing it. Go for it. I think if people want to put the money, want to try and have their own biological children, they should go for it. There are a lot of scary things about adoption even when you make the decision to do it.

MIKE: I don't know how we held it together. I really don't. I think the advice that I would give to anyone who is going through it is the same kind of advice that you give, the same kind of discipline you put on yourself if you go to Las Vegas and you gamble. I go, okay, I can lose two or three hundred dollars. And that's it, and that's how much money I take, and when that's gone, then I'm through for the night. I've had my night's entertainment. If I'm up a couple hundred dollars, that's even better. I think you've got to decide not only financially but emotionally how much you can invest in doing this.

I think Chris and Kate would agree. They spent almost everything they had, all their money and all their hope, but what they did not lose was their vision of life with children, their vision of being parents, being a family.

CHRIS: As amazing as it is, nothing's a sure thing. It was a learning experience. We both learned a lot about who we are. It tests your love, it tests your convictions, and with regard to the science, I remember when Kate had her laparoscopy, I mean, that was difficult, it was painful to watch her being wheeled into the operating room and being put under sedation and then afterward to watch the video!! I'm looking at the inside of my wife's body. It was amazing.
KATE: And science is an amazing thing, and the human body is amazing. IVF is a wonderful thing and it works for many, many people and it gives them what they're looking for. So many people are willing to do it several times either because they have the money . . .
CHRIS: Or the drive.
KATE: It just wasn't for us financially and emotionally. We did it as much as we could do it.

CHRIS: Was it worth it? Absolutely.

KATE: Yes.

CHRIS: Absolutely. We would not be the people we are today without having gone through this experience. (A) It brought up some medical issues with Kate that we were unaware of, so there was that positive aspect. (B) It was character building.

KATE: It certainly . . . the whole experience could hurt some people and their relationships, but I think it only made our relationship stronger. It was always strong and a good relationship anyway, but I think having gone through all that, it just made us closer, and it made us realize what's really important. I will tell you that once we decided to adopt that it was such a weight lifted off my shoulders, and I felt such relief and all of a sudden I was myself again, and I have been ever since we made that decision. If we had not gone through what we went through, we wouldn't have our son, and he is the most beautiful and amazing gift. I don't think we could have made one better if we did it ourselves, because he is so beautiful and such an amazing little boy and truly our gift from God. He must really be what God had planned for us.

CHRIS: I think Kate hit the nail on the head. We just, when you share so many highs and lows together. We were strong, we've always been strong together, but that's where you bare your soul to each other, and we grew together. We were experiencing the same types of things.

KATE: We grieved together.

CHRIS: We did. We grieved, we really did. As crazy as that sounds, we grieved for the child that we never had.

KATE: When I was pregnant, the baby was going to be born in February, and our adopted son was born around the same time, so I felt good about that.

CHRIS: Kate is the mother of my child, and I can't think of anybody who could be a better mom than Kate. That was one of the things, how good she was with children, from the first day I met her, from when I first saw her at school. I can't even tell you how many nieces and nephews she has, she's just so wonderful with children. It was painful to see that this woman was built to be a mother and she wasn't able to do that, and now she is, and that makes me feel so great. We are just so blessed, we really are.

KATE: I always felt, poor Chris, when he met me and married me, he certainly didn't sign on for somebody that couldn't give him a biological child. Coming from, "Oh my God, no way am I ever going to adopt," to, "Sure, I love you and it's okay that you can't have a baby, and we're going to adopt, we're a family, everything's great."

CHRIS: It's called growing up. As we start looking at the way things are put in your path, if maybe our story would inspire somebody that's going through difficulties with IVF to adopt, wow that would certainly make us feel wonderful.

Chris and Kate are still under a heavy debt, but they don't regret spending the money to give it a shot. Even on a teacher's and firefighter's salary, with no outside help, they felt it was worth it.

Tim and Kathy were never shy about their situation, although they may not have told everyone while they were going through it. As journalists, though, they want to tell people of their experiences;

they want people to know that while IVF is behind them, it will always be a part of who they are.

KATHY: People who haven't gone through it don't realize what it took to get our son, so he's just extra special. Now he's just a baby, it's not like he's the IVF baby in the family. It really doesn't come up anymore. It's more about oh he smiled today or he looks like you or what's he doing? It's never about how he got here.

TIM: I'm kind of a blabbermouth, so I don't have a problem talking about this issue, and to me it helped because I talked to a lot of people about it a lot; I told them what was going on, and you couldn't believe the feedback. Everybody knows somebody, it seems, that had this problem. So and so has twins now. You would also hear the bad side. They have no insurance, it's costing them this amount of money. As the stories kind of rolled in, we just all of a sudden realized this is an extreme privilege.

Hey I wanted a baby, you know, I wanted a baby really bad, and dammit I'm going to get one. I'm going to do this!

People have a lot of questions about it. How does it work? Now it's the opposite for me from when we were doing it. People are asking me questions. I'm IVF guy.

Tim should meet Alexandra because if he's "IVF guy," she's "IVF gal." While Alexandra and Peter told no one about their fertility battle, now that they're through it, they tell absolutely everyone, especially since they've had their third child naturally. I've never met two people who are more open and more willing to share their experience just so that they could help others in the same boat. It was a complete switch for them, going from constant silence to constant counsel, but that's what IVF did for them. It forced them to see their situation in a whole new light. What they once cried about, they now laugh about with hints of tears, and who can tell if they are tears of joy or tears of memory. It's an indescribable sense you get from this couple who fought to survive infertility and who are now fighting to survive three children under the age of three. They are all at once solid and frantic, exhilarated and exhausted.

ALEXANDRA: I'd like to start a support group for women because that wasn't there for me. During our fertility battle, I went to a therapist, which helped me. She saved me. I was having a really, really bad anxiety problem, but in a way, it would really have helped me to just bounce it off once a week with strangers and then walk away, not to mom, not take it into my family life, but go somewhere and let off steam and share and that is something that really would've helped me.

I still feel for my particular situation, and really because of the way I am, like once it's out in the open I can't stop talking because I am such an open person, so the fact that I managed to find the strength to keep it, to shut it down, ended up helping me. Because literally if people knew that was my deal, like I am in fertility treatments right now, it's *all* I would have talked about, like at every dinner party, I'd be like, "Let's find a way to get the conversation back to my treatments.

But once I was pregnant, I felt there was nothing to be ashamed of and then I felt like, I immediately started hearing back from people, like well I've got a friend and I told her about you, I was like, "Tell her to call me, tell her to call me!" I mean I just desperately wanted to help other people. I want something to come from my struggle. We ended up with these two unbelievable miracles and that's not enough. I want other women to be helped as well.

PETER: I tend to, well if it comes up, you know if people ask: "Do twins run in the family?" If I'm in the mood to talk, I don't hold back and I want to tell people, but I am not as crazed about it as Alexandra, but I don't have her hormones either.

ALEXANDRA: You have to believe in the science, but then you have to trust the mystery, and that is really hard. You have to say this science is out there, and it works, and it could be a miracle for us, but it might not work. You have to trust that there is just a greater mystery and we don't all get pregnant from in vitro the first time.

Even though the science is the same for everyone, you are on your own path, and you have to find out what this is teaching you about your marriage, what it is teaching you about your greatest fears, how you can learn from that. Infertility is a good lesson that you're not in charge.

AFTERWORD

More than a quarter of a century ago, a doctor somewhere had an idea. If a woman can't get pregnant naturally, why not try this: take her eggs out of her body, put them in a test tube, mix them with her partner's sperm, and then, voilà, put them back into her uterus. Seems simple enough, right? Simple, and yet almost impossible to fathom. These are microscopic organisms, so fragile, so complex, but somebody actually figured out how to do this and changed the courses of a thousand lives. Think of all the people who would have no options without this!

Who could have known a quarter of a century ago that in vitro fertilization would become a billion-dollar business, giving thousands of couples hope that they once would have thought impossible. Think of all the people alive today who wouldn't be alive if it weren't for IVF. To call it a miracle wouldn't do it justice. It is essentially God on earth, if you believe in that kind of thing. It's more than a cure; it's creation!

If that's true, then why do I have such mixed feelings? Why do I get annoyed every time I see a commercial on television for some fertility clinic offering some new cost-efficient deal on IVF? Why do I scoff at the idea that this has become so commonplace? But more important, why do I have such an intense love for my children that is matched only by the intense disdain for how they were brought into this world? I don't mean the procedure: not the drugs, not the doctors, not the lab technicians who make it all possible. I mean the idea, the idea that my children were not conceived in my body, that I didn't make my babies. I just grew them.

I truly admire everyone I interviewed for this book. I have never met such courageous, generous, thoughtful people, and often, in transcribing their words, I felt ashamed at my own. Why don't I marvel at the science? Why don't I shout from the rooftops that IVF is the greatest thing that ever happened to me? Why don't Scott and I ever talk about it? He has none of these feelings, at least he's never said so, and I don't believe he does. Still, while we talk about other people's stories and talk about this book, we rarely go back in time and think about those years of infertility and those months of IVF.

I asked him again recently, as I was writing this afterword, and he said to me, "It's a total disconnect." He actually never thinks about IVF anymore. Instead he marvels at our children, watches their accomplishments, revels in every new word or action, and never for a moment regrets the way they came into this world. He doesn't question for a moment that they are our flesh and blood. He even sounded somewhat annoyed at my questions. "Why do you even think about it?" he says. "We are the luckiest people. We were given such a gift. Why can't you see that?"

I do see that. I really do. But here's the thing: every man gives his sperm away to create a child. Whether it's IVF or just plain old sex, the sperm leaves a man's body and goes somewhere else to become an embryo. That's not so for a woman. A woman not only grows a child in her body, she creates it there. She gives it life.

Trust me, I am no nature lover. I grew up in the middle of New York City, and I wasn't big on going to Central Park. I can fill my body with high-fructose corn syrup on a daily basis, breathe in big-city smog, and spend hours every evening staring at sitcoms instead of gazing at the stars, and yet the fact that my children were not conceived naturally bothers the hell out of me. I did not give my children life inside my body, and to me, thankless as that sounds, therein is the loss.

Do I regret doing IVF? No, absolutely not. Do I regret that it was our only option? Yes. But I also know that we could have waited and tried for a few more years and maybe conceived a child naturally. That wasn't the answer either. I couldn't wait. I couldn't deal with not knowing our fate as a family.

I keep thinking how strange it is that none of the people I interviewed expressed these same feelings, but I wonder if perhaps it isn't something too personal to say out loud. I think all of us, no matter our religious beliefs or our faith in humanity, all of us somehow want to feel connected to something higher, and for a woman, to create life inside her own body, that is the connection to something higher.

I spend my days in the hackneyed, overdramatized world of TV news and I walk down busy streets where people don't look at each other. I come home to a world of expectations of parenthood: Are my kids doing the right things, saying the right things for their age? Did I enroll them in the right preschool? Is my nanny intellectually stimulating enough? Am I teaching my children right from wrong? Am I loving them enough? Am I loving them too much?

It's easy to get caught up in all of that and lose sight of what's really important: We made children when the odds were clearly against us. We got something that some people believe we don't deserve, something beyond all value, something beyond even the word, "gift." Still, it took me a long time to feel the bond of motherhood with my children. The connection was not immediately there, and perhaps that was IVF, perhaps it was infertility in general.

I believe that couples who spend years battling infertility are often unprepared for success, unprepared for actually having children. Infertility involves so much research, so much stress, so much discussion, and so much learning, that couples are often too exhausted, too talked out or in too much disbelief to do all the research and stressing and expending of all the energy that a normal potential parent does in the months before a child arrives. I know I was completely unprepared for parenthood, never mind twins. I can cite you chapter and verse on fertility treatment ratios and tell you umpteen stories of umpteen couples in umpteen struggles, but I had never changed a diaper before my children arrived. I didn't read the books, Scott and I didn't discuss philosophies of parenting, and most important I didn't prepare myself for motherhood.

When my twins arrived, I felt as if I were handed these tiny, needy things that I knew nothing about. I was scared for their survival and my own. I know, it's unfair to generalize, given my horrific last week of pregnancy and the emergency circumstances of their birth, but I have to admit I did not feel that immediate connection that all those exhausted, sweaty women seem to exude when you see them on TV just after giving birth, baby cupped in their arms as if it were still a part of their body. I never did get that.

Again, I realize that there are plenty of parents out there who conceived naturally and experienced the same emotions I did. They may not be unique to IVF parents, but from the research I, and others, have done I do believe that these emotions can be triggered and/or exacerbated by IVF. I write this so that some other potential mother out there might be a little more prepared than I was for the unique emotional aftereffects of IVF. For some people, conception may be the end of the cycle of infertility; IVF may be a finite process that becomes a fond memory for some, but it's not that way for everyone. And that's okay.

There is no shame in admitting that a scientific process that results in something as unscientific as a human soul can be so hard to reconcile. Someone invaded my body and took my most valuable possessions, my eggs. Yes, that person did something miraculous with those eggs and gave me back the gift I had longed for, but it does change something, something that has absolutely, positively nothing to do with the unimaginably beautiful children I tuck into bed every evening.

I struggled a long time to understand why I have these feelings and kept coming back to the same argument in my head: I love my children with all my heart. I worry and wonder about them just like every other mother. I watch them, listen to them, hang on their every gurgle and grunt. If they're congested, I can't breathe. If they feel pain in their flesh, I feel it in my bones. So what's missing in my children? The answer is nothing, absolutely nothing. This is not about them.

This is about me, me and IVF and my feelings of inadequacy that I was unable to create life on my own, that I could not be "normal." It's about fear, irrational fears of some mistake in a laboratory or some as-yet unknown side effect of the science, or other consequences my noxious imagination hasn't conjured yet. Shame on me for mixing that up with my children, shame on me for blaming my husband for my own fears, and shame on me for letting those feelings rob me of the joys of motherhood.

It's time to let it go.

Twenty months after my children were born, I went on my first business trip away from home. I was terrified about how much I would miss them, more terrified that they would be safe while I was away. Of course I trust my husband to take care of them, but like every other crazy Jewish mother, I felt that my children are obviously only safe when I am within a taxi-able distance.

I brought pictures with me, but for some reason I was afraid to look at the pictures for the first two days I was away. I don't know, maybe I thought seeing the pictures would make me miss them so much I wouldn't be able to function. But it was something different; strangely, in those first days, it seemed almost as if the whole thing, infertility, IVF, my pregnancy, the first year of raising these little twins, all of it seemed like a dream.

Finally, on the second night, I pulled the pictures out of their envelope and lined them up on the night table. And there it was. Suddenly I saw something that startled me. It was something I had really never seen before. It only took one look, but there it was, plain as day. I saw myself, and I saw Scott. In the faces of these giggly, drooling toddlers, there we were.

Where did we come from? Why had I never seen it before? Why did I have to leave in order to come back to the truth, a truth I had sought for almost two years? These are my children. My husband and I created them, and if we needed a little help to do that, then that is just fine. Something in those pictures said to me, "It's time to say thank you and move on." Why? Because if I don't, then I am going to miss so much, so much that Scott is reveling in without me. Time spent stressing over science and self is now time wasted. It took me a long time to see that, too long, but I see that now. How could I miss it when it was staring right back at me from those pictures on my night table?

If science can save life, then science can create life, and there's nothing unnatural about it. Yes, my children traveled through needles, soaked in stuff that was made in a laboratory, and became who and what they are in a dish, before they finally came to rest inside me. And that's okay. A symphony is made of wood and metal and the work of fingers and lungs, but the resulting music is no less mysterious, natural nor ethereal than the looks of joy and wonder deep inside my children's eyes.

Science is an amazing thing, and doctors are amazing people. In vitro fertilization is nothing short of a profound accomplishment. Life under glass. Something so precious in something so fragile that creates something so strong. From science came souls. From hope came human beings. From me and from Scott, came Noah and Madeline. Finally, a family.

INDEX